Dirty Sanchez's Guide to
BUCK NASTY SEX

Dirty Sanchez's Guide to
BUCK NASTY SEX

Copyright © 2010 Ulysses Press and its licensors. All rights reserved under International and Pan-American Copyright Conventions, including the right to reproduce this book or portions thereof in any form whatsoever, except for use by a reviewer in connection with a review.

Published by: Amorata Press,
an imprint of Ulysses Press
P.O. Box 3440
Berkeley, CA 94703
www.amoratapress.com

ISBN13: 978-1-56975-720-8
Library of Congress Control Number: 2009924089

Printed in the United States by Bang Printing

10 9 8 7 6 5

Acquisitions editor: Nick Denton-Brown
Managing editor: Claire Chun
Editors: Lily Chou, Emma Silvers, Lauren Harrison, Elyce Petker
Production: Abigail Reser
Design and layout: Wade Nights

Distributed by Publishers Group West

PUBLISHER'S NOTE: This book is a parody and is offered for the entertainment and amusement of the reader. Any reader who might decide to "do the undoable" by trying to imitate the outlandish positions and practices described here is strongly cautioned to beware of the physical injuries and sexually transmitted diseases that may result. You do so at your own risk!

CONTENTS

Introduction
11

Cincinnati Bow Tie
12

Space Docking
22

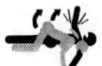
Alligator Fuckhouse
14

Birmingham Booty Call
24

Hot Lips Houlihan
16

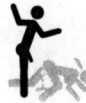
Cherry Cream Pie
26

Boston Pancake
18

Dirty Gas Pump
28

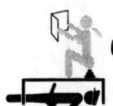
Glass-Bottom Boat
20

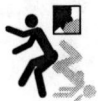
Two Cats in the Bathtub
30

The Stranger
32

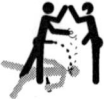 **Abe Lincoln**
46

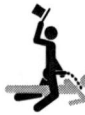 **Pearl Necklace**
34

 Alabama Hot Pocket
48

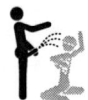 **Golden Shower**
36

 Hot Lunch
50

 Strawberry Shortcake
38

 Reverse Blumpkin
52

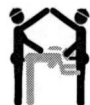 **Eiffel Tower**
40

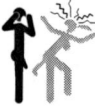 **Pink Sock**
54

 Tea Bag
42

 Cleveland Steamer
56

 Chili Dog
44

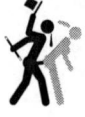 **Houdini**
58

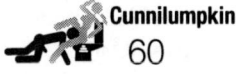 **Cunnilumpkin**
60

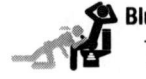 **Blumpkin**
74

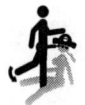 **Angry Pirate**
62

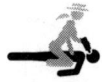 **Mommy Dearest**
76

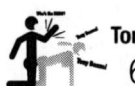 **Tony Danza**
64

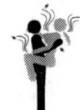 **Burning Man**
78

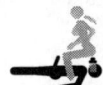 **Hot Carl**
66

 Camel Hump
80

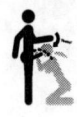 **Angry Dragon**
68

 Deep-Sea Fishing
82

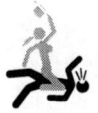 **Bronco**
70

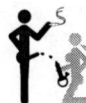 **Highball**
84

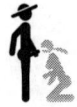 **Dirty Sanchez**
72

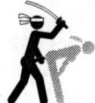 **Kamikaze**
86

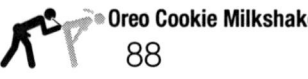 **Oreo Cookie Milkshake** 88

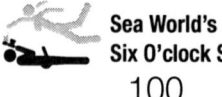 **Sea World's Six O'clock Show** 100

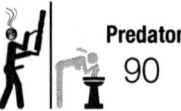 **Predator** 90

 **Speed Baggin'** 102

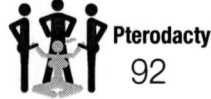 **Pterodactyl** 92

 **Superman** 104

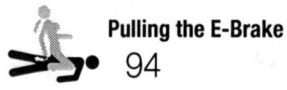 **Pulling the E-Brake** 94

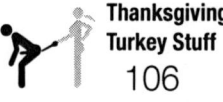 **Thanksgiving Turkey Stuff** 106

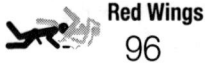 **Red Wings** 96

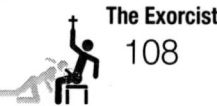 **The Exorcist** 108

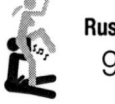 **Rusty Tuba** 98

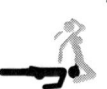 **The Last Unicorn** 110

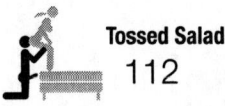 **Tossed Salad** 112

 **Rusty Trombone** 122

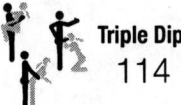 **Triple Dip** 114

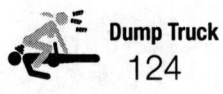 **Dump Truck** 124

 **Vampire Tea Bag** 116

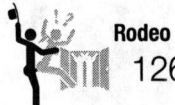 **Rodeo** 126

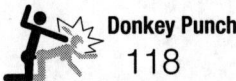 **Donkey Punch** 118

About the Author 128

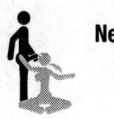 **New Delhi Dot** 120

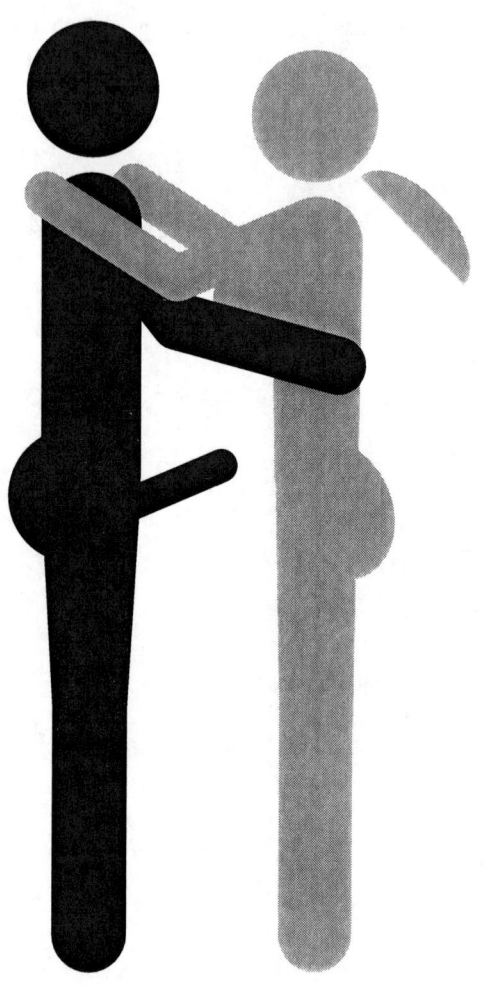

INTRODUCTION

There is sex, there's adventurous sex and then there's mind-blowing, dirty, nasty sex. This is the sex that most partners never get to experience due to natural hygienic concerns, physical fears and subtle sexual inhibition. This is the type of love-making that uses every sense, body movement and slightly disturbing act imaginable to explore the bounds of human sexuality. Going beyond novice acts like petting, caressing, kissing and penetrating, this guide will show you how to use every part of your body to turn an erotic encounter into an experience you will never forget—no matter how hard you try.

So set aside what you think you know about sex and let us guide you into an amazing new world of orgasmic love-making.

CINCINNATI BOW TIE
Cincinnatus cavus

Commonly referred to as "reverse titty fucking," the derivation comes from the bow tie shape of the male's testicles as they rest flayed upon his partner's neck. The classic finish to the position is the "double breast" with pearl buttons.

Props: Martini glass, evening gloves, elegant cigarette holder.

Hot Tip: Nothing says formal evening wear like a well shorn bow tie; the woolly bow tie, popular during the 1970s, has yet to come back into fashion.

Degree of Difficulty

Degree of Nastiness

"I married him because I thought he was a gentleman, but when he dazzled me with a beautiful Cincinnati Bow Tie, I realized just how fabulous he really is."

Myrtle
Philanthropist
New York, New York

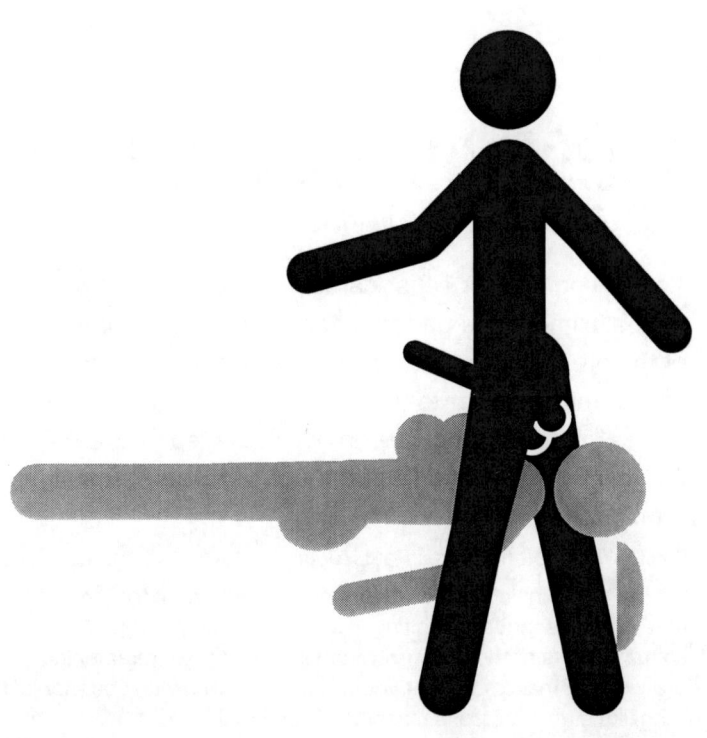

☐ Did It.

Date: ___/___/___   Partner: _____

My Personal Enjoyment (1-10): ☐   My Partner's Enjoyment (1-10): ☐

Comment: _____
_____
_____

CINCINNATI BOW TIE

ALLIGATOR FUCKHOUSE
Conglomero crocodylus

An exciting end for either participant. At the point of mutual climax, one partner bites down on the corner of the other's neck, near the shoulder, and initiates a "death roll"—similar to the efficient hunting technique of an alligator or crocodile, in which the reptile breaks its victim's bones and flesh through vigorous, sensual rotations.

Props: Wide, soft mattress; Paul Hogan or Steve Irwin cutout.

Hot Tip: When initiating the "death roll," it's important to remember that while this move is exciting, it's also extremely dangerous. With so many parts of the body entwined and your teeth threatening to draw blood, make sure that your partner is rolling with you, not just lying like a dead carcass mashed under a rock.

Degree of Difficulty

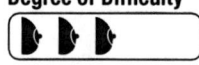

Degree of Nastiness

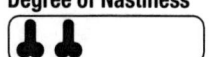

> *"Nethin' prepares me for the great thrill of an Alligator Fuckhouse after an hour of love-making. Daisy is a big girl, 6'1" and heavy as a truck, so when she starts rolling me, I know that our climax is going to be anything but dull. The bleeding usually stops within an hour, and the occasional broken rib is just a small price to pay."*
>
> Sam
> Outdoorsman
> Perth, Australia

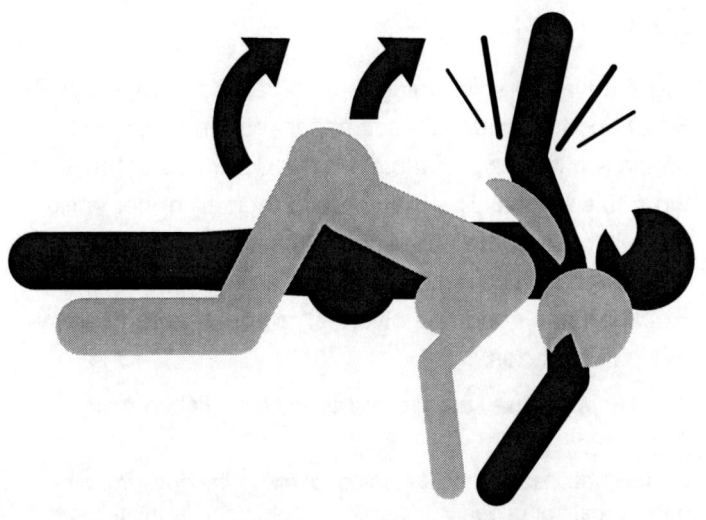

☐ Did It.

Date: ___/___/___   Partner: _____

My Personal
Enjoyment (1-10): ☐

My Partner's
Enjoyment (1-10): ☐

Comment: _____
_____
_____

ALLIGATOR FUCKHOUSE

HOT LIPS HOULIHAN
Ferveo labia

A great way to spice things up in the bedroom — literally. Before coitus, pour Tabasco sauce (habanero or "rooster" sauce are both acceptable) on the outer lips of the woman's vagina. The man should then enter her while the full force of the hot sauce takes effect. Originally conceived and coined in the Louisiana bayou, Hot Lips Houlihan has become universally popular among spicy-food aficionados.

Props: Pepper-based hot sauce, ice-cold bath, cold compress, safety word.

Hot Tip: Water does almost nothing to relieve the body from the burning pain of peppers. Instead of a cold bath, fill the tub with cool milk to neutralize the burn.

Degree of Difficulty

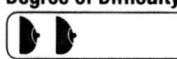

Degree of Nastiness

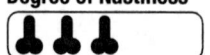

> "We loves us some spicy food. But taking that south-of-the-border taste, well, south of the border really heated up the old bedroom. Nothing will make you as frisky as second-degree burns."
>
> *Carl*
> *Alligator farmer*
> *Baton Rouge, Louisiana*

DIRTY SANCHEZ'S GUIDE TO BUCK NASTY SEX

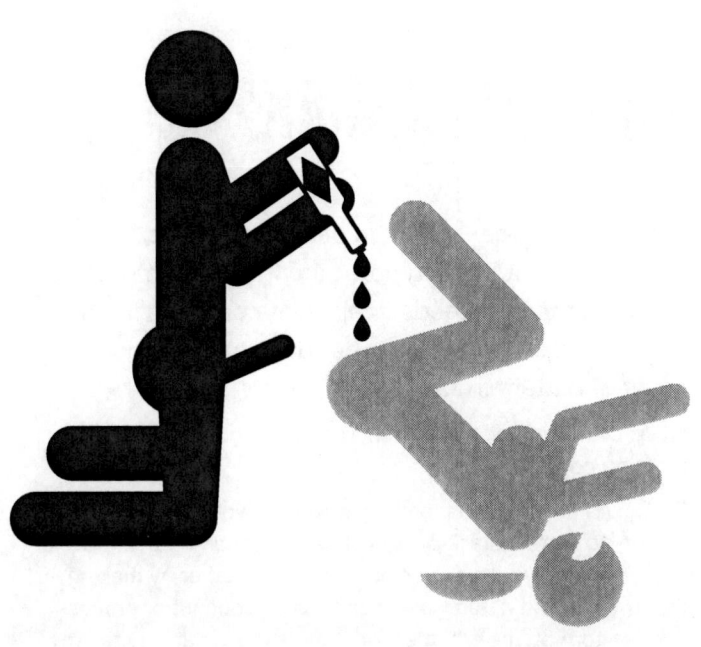

☐ Did It.

Date: ___/___/___ Partner: _____

My Personal Enjoyment (1-10): ⬜   My Partner's Enjoyment (1-10): ⬜

Comment: _____
_____
_____

HOT LIPS HOULIHAN

BOSTON PANCAKE
Botolph crustum

Just before climax, the man defecates on the woman's chest, patting down the fresh pile into a flat cake. He then proceeds to ejaculate onto the freshly pressed cake, mimicking a hot dash of syrup on a stack of buttermilks.

Props: Drawn butter, cup of coffee, side of homefries, morning paper.

Hot Tip: As any breakfast enthusiast will tell you, consistency is the key to a great stack of pancakes. Before giving this move a go, make sure you're not going to spoil the batter by making it too runny. Avoid natural laxatives such as coconut or prunes. A bit of corn on the cob the night before is a great way to turn this delicacy into sumptuous "corn fritters."

Degree of Difficulty

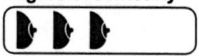

Degree of Nastiness

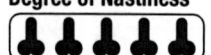

> *"It took me and my wife years to get the Boston Pancake right. I have IBS, and could never quite get the consistency right. I found the less water I drink the night before, the more solid it turns out. But get a good spatula, the lumps can be difficult."*
>
> Phil
> Short order cook
> Houston, Texas

DIRTY SANCHEZ'S GUIDE TO BUCK NASTY SEX

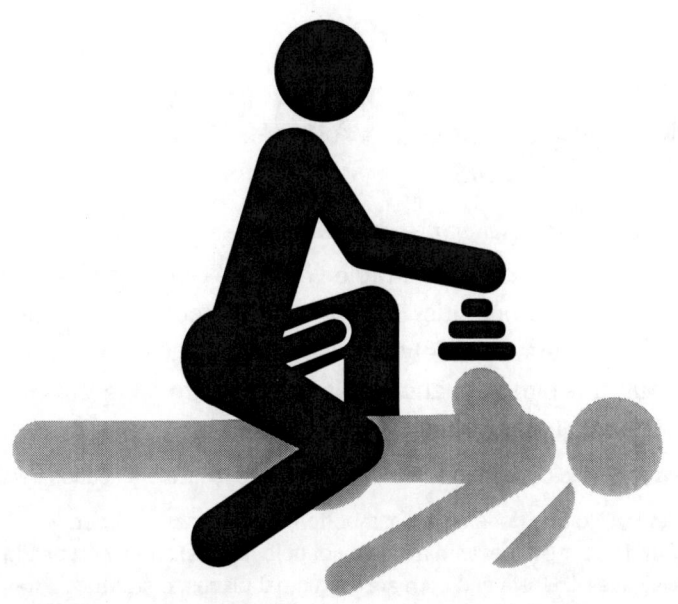

☐ Did It.

Date: ___/___/___   Partner: _____

My Personal
Enjoyment (1-10): ⬜   My Partner's
Enjoyment (1-10): ⬜

Comment: _____
_____
_____

BOSTON PANCAKE

GLASS-BOTTOM BOAT
Traba crystalis

In this perfect addition to foreplay, one partner lies beneath a glass coffee table while the other squats above it and unloads. Like viewing the colorful sea life from the relative safety and serenity of a glass-bottom boat, this simple maneuver is not only arousing but biologically tantalizing.

Props: Glass coffee table, Windex, laminated fecal identification card.

Hot Tip: No one goes on a glass-bottom boat to stare at trout. Dazzle your partner with a medley of color and texture by preparing well ahead. Beets and corn are both great places to start.

Degree of Difficulty

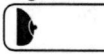

Degree of Nastiness

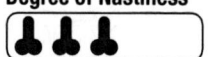

> *"I've been to Hawaii. I've seen all of those fish—it's what every tourist does. It's neat and all, but never blew me away. But getting to see my Bobby in action, seeing that magical human process going on in front of me... well, I just felt like a science student all over again."*
>
> Barbara
> Telemarketer
> Indianapolis, Indiana

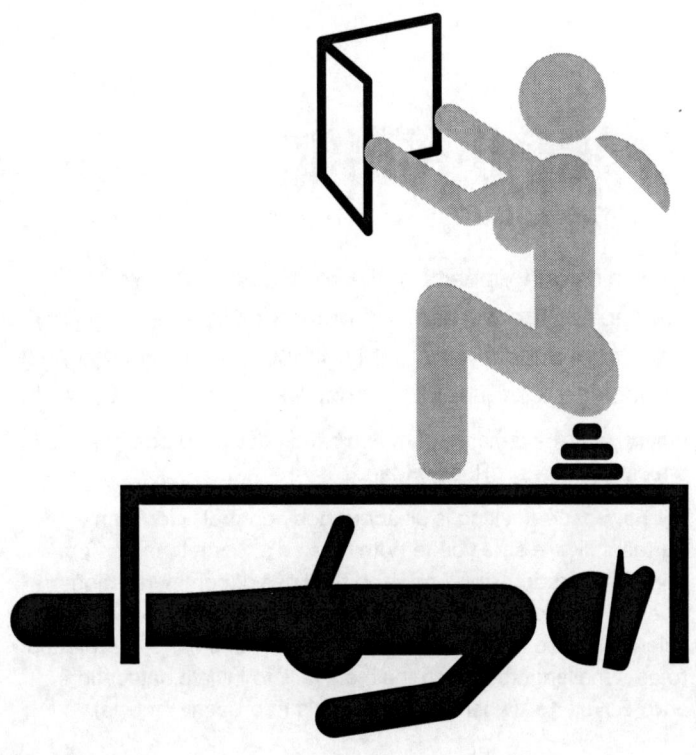

☐ Did It.

Date: ___/___/___   Partner: _____

My Personal Enjoyment (1-10): ☐   My Partner's Enjoyment (1-10): ☐

Comment: _____
_____
_____

GLASS-BOTTOM BOAT

SPACE DOCKING
Incursio astrum

Mid-missionary position, the man pulls out, turns his back to the woman and defecates into her vagina. This maneuver is remarkably difficult, hence the likeness to docking a shuttle into a space station at 17,000 mph.

Props: Hand-held mirror, communication device, procedure checklist, copy of "Rocket Man."

Hot Tip: Space docking is all about body control—for both partners. Make sure you're both relaxed and stretched before commencing docking. And keep the lines of communication open or accidents can occur. After all, this is pretty much rocket science. Failed attempts are extremely common and are referred to as "Challengers" (when the male fails to initiate defecation) and "Soyuz-1s" (when the female fails to properly receive).

Degree of Difficulty

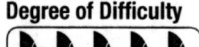

Degree of Nastiness

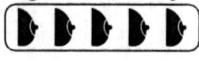

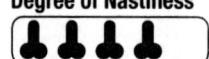

"I have a huge space-travel fetish and this is just like 'one small drop for [a] man, one giant orgasm for mankind.'"
"Buzz"
Aerospace technician
Pasadena, California

DIRTY SANCHEZ'S GUIDE TO BUCK NASTY SEX

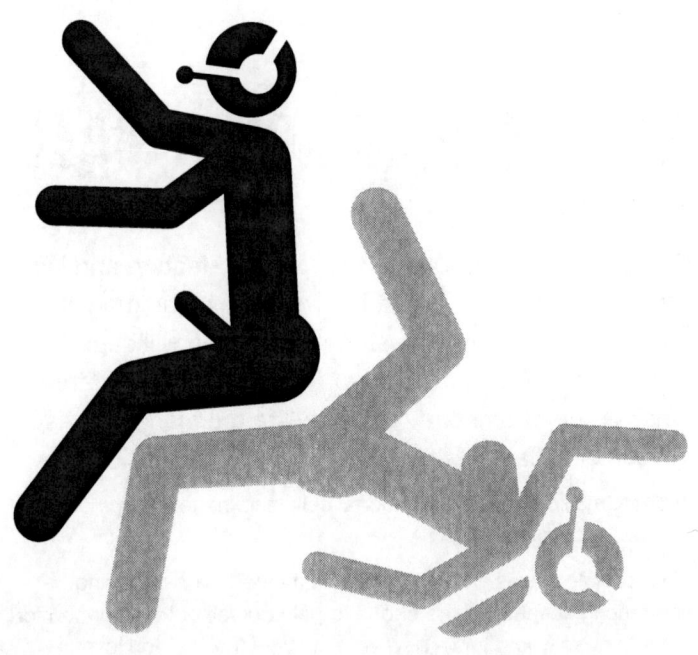

☐ Did It.

Date: ___/___/___   Partner: _____

My Personal
Enjoyment (1-10): ☐

My Partner's
Enjoyment (1-10): ☐

Comment: _____
_____
_____

SPACE DOCKING

BIRMINGHAM BOOTY CALL
Dico lino

Set a cellular telephone to the "vibrate" feature and insert into the man's rectum just before climax. The man should then call the phone. The strong vibrations will cause the man to release the phone. The woman should then answer the phone and "talk dirty" to the man while he gives her a "facial."

Props: Small cell phone; additional cell, landline telephone or Skype; Astroglide.

Hot Tip: Role play is always fun play in the bedroom. Try using interesting accents on the phone to get yourself out of your comfort zone. You may just find a new voracity with the one you love.

Degree of Difficulty

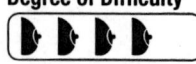

Degree of Nastiness

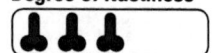

> "The long distance was hard. For a year we had phone sex, Skype sex, but no physical connection. When we finally found ourselves together, we didn't know how to behave. The Birmingham Booty Call allowed us to find the perfect melding of what we knew and what we didn't."
>
> *Faith*
> *Student*
> *Los Angeles, California*

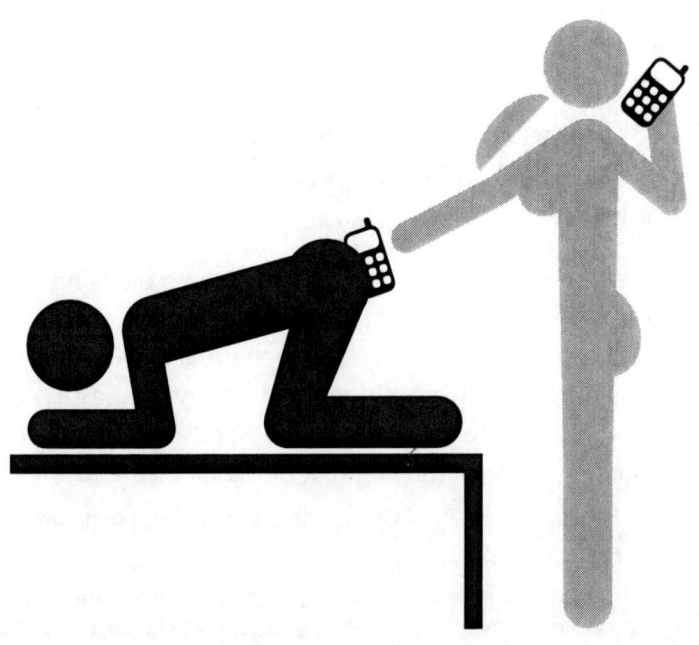

☐ Did It.

Date: ___/___/___   Partner: _____

My Personal
Enjoyment (1-10): ☐   My Partner's
Enjoyment (1-10): ☐

Comment: _____
_____
_____

BIRMINGHAM BOOTY CALL

CHERRY CREAM PIE
Strages

An iron-infused twist on the classic "cream pie," the Cherry Cream Pie is a tantalizing finish for any couple having sex during the woman's menstrual cycle. After ejaculating inside his partner, the man watches as the woman expels the seed along with her period blood, creating a visually stunning mix of reds, pinks and white.

Props: 6" pie tin, Easy-Bake Oven, video camera, extra tampons.

Hot Tip: Follow the old adage, "The fresher the cherries, the better the pie." Always complete your cherry cream pie early in the woman's cycle, when her period is less spotty and metallic in taste.

Degree of Difficulty
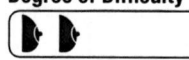

Degree of Nastiness
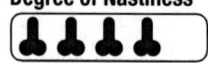

"Mmmm, pie."

Dave
Insurance salesman
San Diego, California

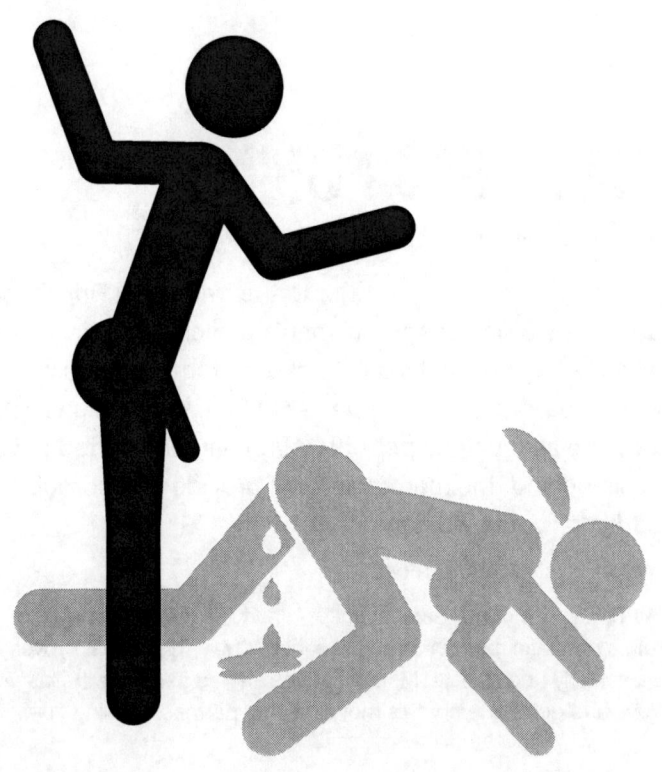

☐ Did It.

Date: ___/___/___   Partner: _____

My Personal
Enjoyment (1-10): ☐   My Partner's
Enjoyment (1-10): ☐

Comment: _____
_____
_____

CHERRY CREAM PIE

DIRTY GAS PUMP
Immunda ientaculum

Adding a little Southern twist to the traditional British tea bag, the woman brings the man's testicles into her mouth while facing his backside. As she performs a handjob while "tea-bagging" (see page 42) him, the man should flatulate as much as possible. With her face buried deep in his behind, the man's wind will provide an odorous addition for the woman.

Props: Flavorful, ethnic meal.

Hot Tip: An accidental defecation, or "shart," is the easiest way to ruin a romantic moment in any situation, but in this case it proves particularly unfortunate. Mind what you've had to eat for the last few days and don't attempt this move if either partner is feeling flu-y.

Degree of Difficulty

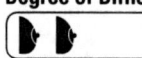

Degree of Nastiness

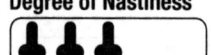

> *"I think the key to surviving a Dirty Gas Pump is breath control. Eventually you learn when to breathe through the nose, alternating with removing the balls, for deep breaths through the mouth. It's not hard, but until you get the hang of it, it's not pleasant."*
>
> *Olga*
> *Lamaze coach*
> *Washington, D.C.*

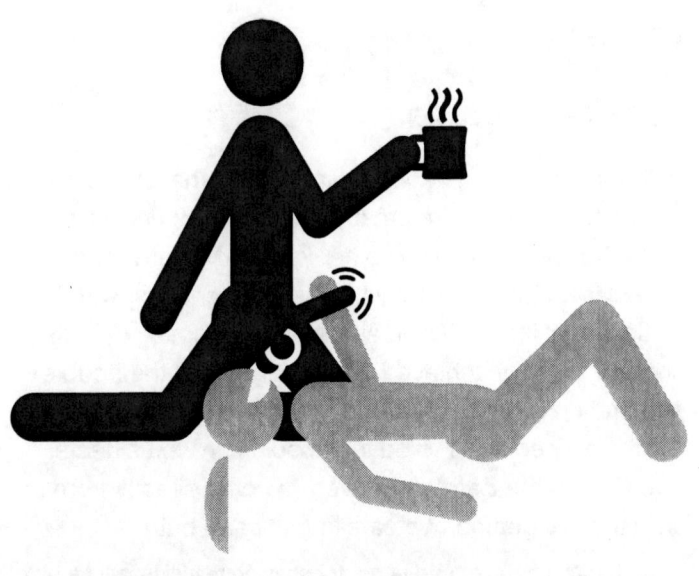

☐ Did It.

Date: ___/___/___   Partner: _____

My Personal Enjoyment (1-10): ☐   My Partner's Enjoyment (1-10): ☐

Comment: _____
_____
_____

DIRTY GAS PUMP

TWO CATS IN THE BATHTUB
Duae feles lavatio

With the woman on her back and legs in the air, the man begins by taking a firm grasp of his testicles and then tenderly inserting them into her vagina. Maneuvering carefully, he then inserts his penis into her anus, with his testicles still inside. While either partner climaxing in this position is rarely achieved, the sheer thrill of the double penetration is arousing for both people. Considered by most sex specialists to be the absolute in sexual feats, Two Cats in the Bathtub derives its name directly from the challenge of getting two cats into a warm bath.

Props: Lubricant, razor and lather for shaving testicles, a little bit of flexibility and courage.

Hot Tip: If you can successfully complete this position to the point of climax, tell everyone. You are amazing.

Degree of Difficulty

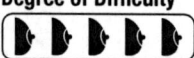

Degree of Nastiness

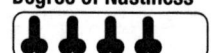

"After months of trying, we finally hit the Two Cats in the Bathtub perfectly. He proposed right afterward. It was the most romantic experience of my life."

Samantha
Fashion consultant
Hoboken, New Jersey

DIRTY SANCHEZ'S GUIDE TO BUCK NASTY SEX

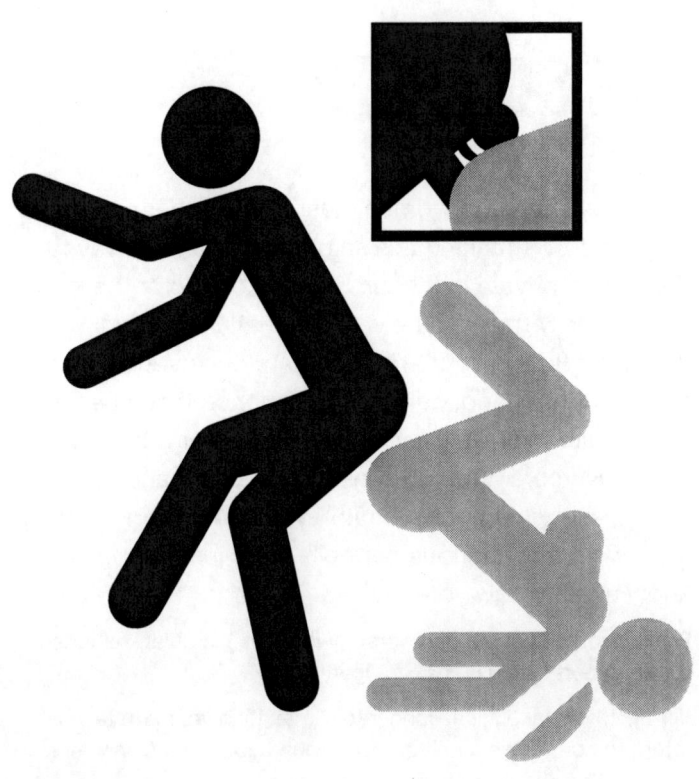

☐ Did It.

Date: ___/___/___ Partner: _____

My Personal
Enjoyment (1-10): ☐   My Partner's
Enjoyment (1-10): ☐

Comment: _____
_____
_____

TWO CATS IN THE BATH TUB

THE STRANGER
Peregrinus

Almost all men and women masturbate either sitting or lying down, making this solo move a natural way to spice up a private half hour. Sit or lie on top of the hand you normally masturbate with, dramatically reducing the blood flow in your arm. For men, once you've lost feeling in that hand, dab on some lubricant and begin to masturbate. Women can start with fingers or a toy—the choice is yours. With no sensation in your hand (but feeling everything down south), you can imagine getting frisky with a mysterious partner—who just happens to know exactly how you like it!

Props: Lubricant; toys; pornography (optional); a quiet, secluded locale; Albert Camus' *The Stranger*.

Hot Tip: If you take a little longer to climax than your arm takes to return to normal, tie a belt or rope around your arm. Consider it auto-erotic asphyxiation for beginners.

Degree of Difficulty

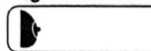

Degree of Nastiness

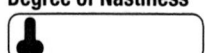

> "I haven't had a partner for some time. And I never had the money or desire to invest in sex toys or call girls. The Stranger really is the next best thing to getting it for real."
>
> *Dan*
> *Auto mechanic*
> *Detroit, Michigan*

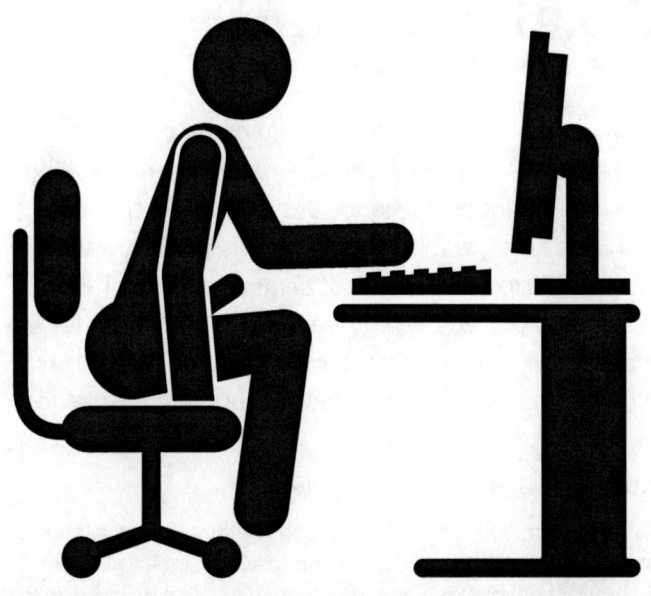

☐ Did It.

Date: ___/___/___   Partner: _____

My Personal Enjoyment (1-10): ☐   My Partner's Enjoyment (1-10): ☐

Comment: _____
_____
_____

THE STRANGER

PEARL NECKLACE
Peractio sumptuosus

Most women ask themselves one question, "Spit or swallow?" Few ever consider this elegant, exciting finale to a successful hand- or blowjob. As the man ejaculates, the woman should pull his penis toward her neck and allow the beads of semen to form a milky, steaming necklace—a guaranteed jaw-dropper for any man. Small variations are key. Try concluding a morning blowjob this way, often called "giving him a 'Breakfast at Tiffany's.'"

Props: Prom dress, champagne flute.

Hot Tips: Men, you may not be able to tell the difference between pear, button or drop pearls, but your partner surely will. Work on your crafting technique ahead of time, delivering delicate dollops of semen onto a practice sheet. For those who become especially proficient "jewelers," try your hand at giving your partner a necklace and crowning tiara with the same spray.

Degree of Difficulty

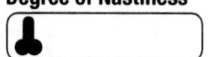

Degree of Nastiness

> "There is nothing, and I mean nothing, like a man who can deliver a perfect pearl necklace. Holding and releasing. The warm beads evenly spaced. The faint aroma. The matching earrings."
>
> *Catherine*
> *Socialite*
> *New York, New York*

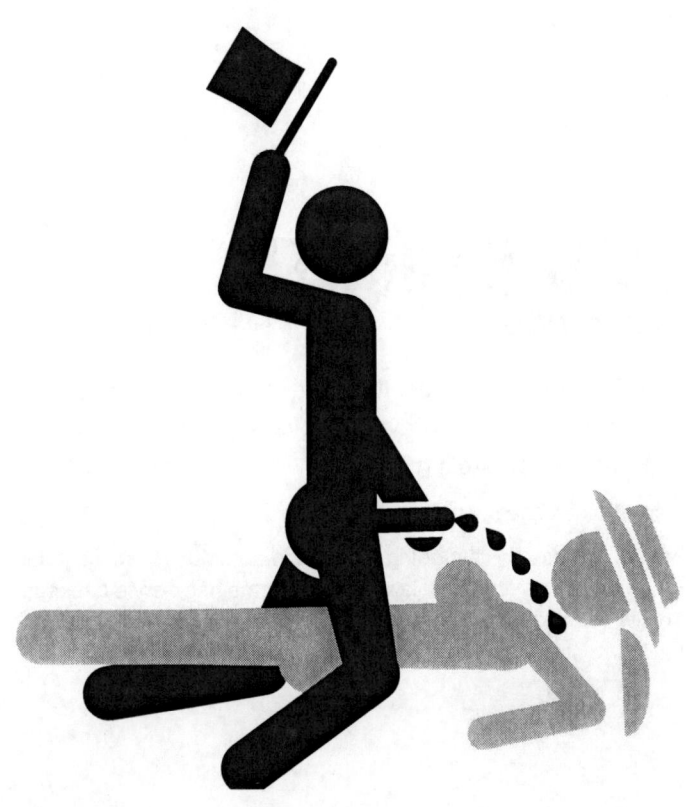

☐ Did It.

Date: ___/___/___ Partner: _____

My Personal Enjoyment (1-10): ☐   My Partner's Enjoyment (1-10): ☐

Comment: _____
_____
_____

PEARL NECKLACE

GOLDEN SHOWER
Mictus pluvia

The simplest of fetishes, the Golden Shower involves one partner simply spraying a lover or friend with the warm drops of one's micturition.

Props: Plastic sheet, sponges.

Hot Tip: To keep the fun going longer and continue to "make it rain," try enjoying this fetish while wearing a Camelback-style backpack. This will allow you access to a continuous stream of liquid without having to stop for water breaks.

Degree of Difficulty

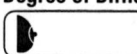

Degree of Nastiness

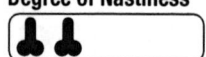

> "Urine has never gotten the attention it deserves in the sexual world. Sure, it's great for expelling waste, but did you know that it's also great for spraying on teen girls in order to obtain an erection?"
>
> R. Kelly
> Musician
> Chicago, Illinois

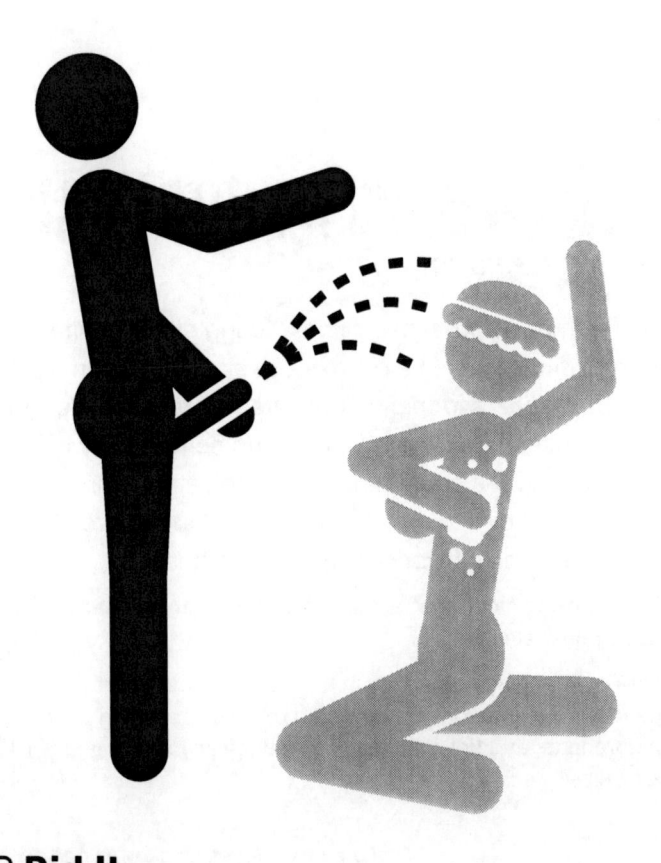

☐ **Did It.**

Date: ___/___/___   Partner: _____

My Personal
Enjoyment (1-10): ☐   My Partner's
Enjoyment (1-10): ☐

Comment: _____
_____
_____

GOLDEN SHOWER

STRAWBERRY SHORTCAKE
Spermae sanguinis

As the man approaches climax during either genital or oral intercourse, he pulls out to ejaculate upon his partner's face and then immediately punches his partner in the nose, thus causing blood and semen to swirl upon his lover's countenance in a delectable mixture reminiscent of the strawberries and whipped cream from everyone's favorite summertime dessert.

Props: Boxing glove, first-aid kit, whipped cream and strawberries to demonstrate intent.

Hot Tip: Punching somebody in the face can really hurt your hand. So be sure to wrap up with a towel or punching glove beforehand, and have ice ready to reduce any swelling in your knuckles afterward.

Degree of Difficulty

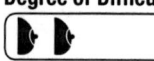

Degree of Nastiness

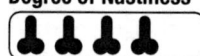

> *"My boyfriend loves Donkey Punching me in the back of the head, but it's so demeaning for me not to make love face to face. It makes me feel like a piece of meat. So instead we started Strawberry Shortcaking. I get to look him in the eyes, and he gets to punch me in the face."*
>
> *Angie*
> *Customer service specialist*
> *Jacksonville, Florida*

DIRTY SANCHEZ'S GUIDE TO BUCK NASTY SEX

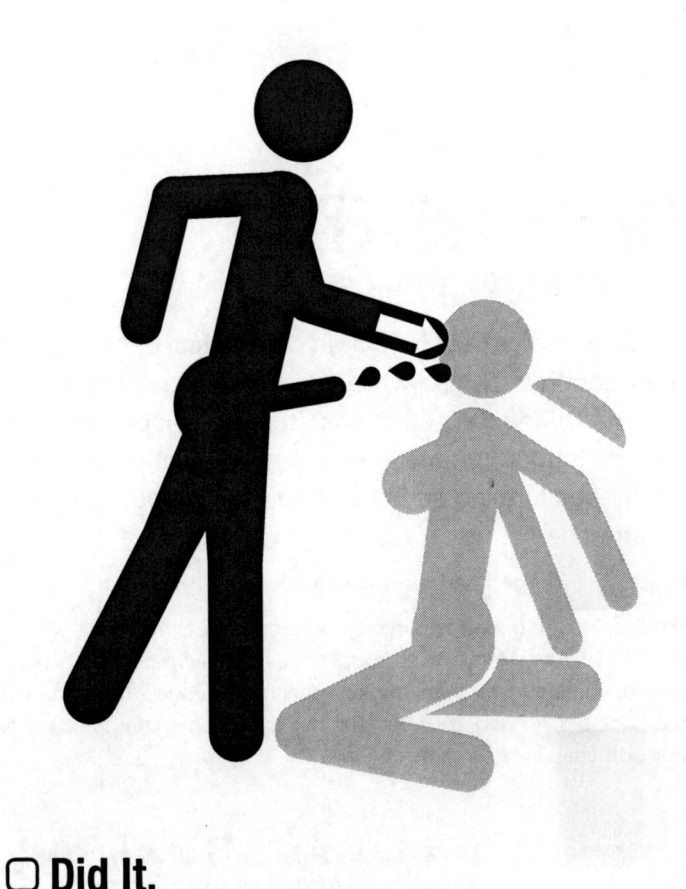

☐ Did It.

Date: ___/___/___   Partner: _____

My Personal
Enjoyment (1-10): ☐   My Partner's
Enjoyment (1-10): ☐

Comment: _____
_____
_____

STRAWBERRY SHORTCAKE

EIFFEL TOWER
Concelebratio veneriis

In this group sex act, one man penetrates, or "doggies," a woman from behind while another gets a blowjob in front. During their exertions, the men — jubilant over their good fortune — reach up and high-five each other, thus forming an Eiffel Tower–like shape with their outstretched arms.

Props: Multi-orificed partner, male friend.

Hot Tip: Though tempting, never combine the Donkey Punch with the Eiffel Tower. Many tower fronts have lost their penises when over-exuberant tower rears donkey-punch the connecting woman in the back of the head, thus causing her to bite down hard and sever any soft flesh in her mouth.

Degree of Difficulty

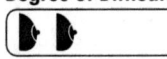

Degree of Nastiness

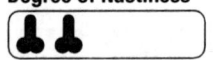

"I use the Eiffel Tower on all my teams to build teamwork and camaraderie. If a couple of my players start fighting, I'll grab the waterboy and tell him to bend over and start sucking until my players learn to work together as a team. When that high-five happens, I know it's all coming together."

Rick
Basketball coach
Salt Lake City, Utah

DIRTY SANCHEZ'S GUIDE TO BUCK NASTY SEX

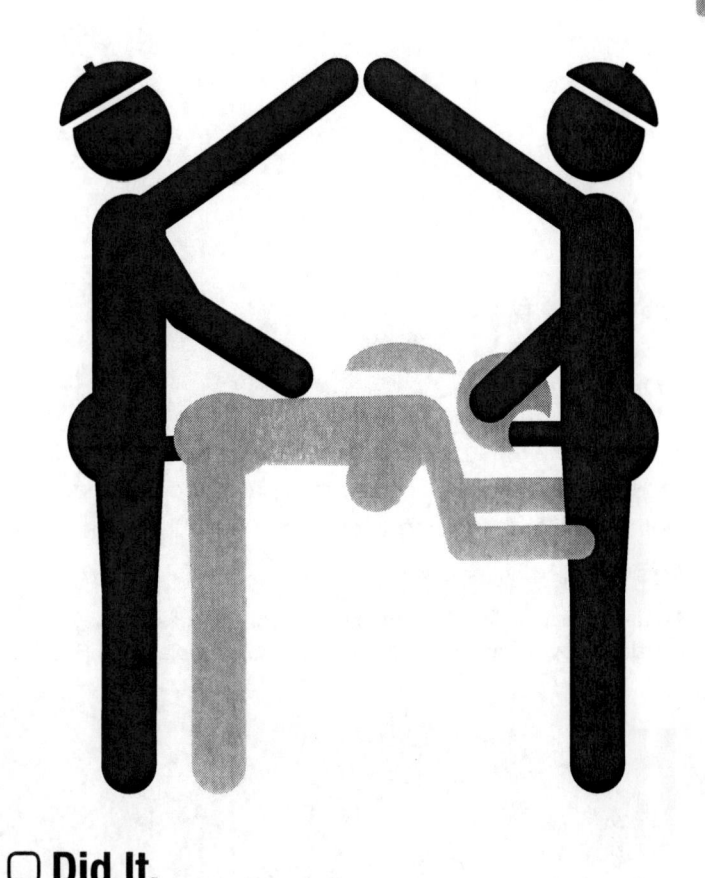

☐ Did It.

Date: ___/___/___ Partner: _____

My Personal
Enjoyment (1-10): ☐

My Partner's
Enjoyment (1-10): ☐

Comment: _____
_____
_____

EIFFEL TOWER

TEA BAG
Coleus gustatus

In this simple fetish, the man repeatedly dips his testicles into the open mouth of his lover or passed-out friend, in a motion similar to dipping a tea bag into a cup of hot water.

Props: Large, hairy testicles.

Hot Tip: Advanced Tea Baggers can smear their balls with feces in order to give their lover the extra-special Chocolate Tea Bag.

Degree of Difficulty

Degree of Nastiness

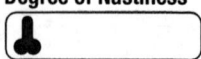

> "Republicans want to sully the good name of the Tea Bag by associating it with tax revolt parties. But this aggression will not stand. We must demand that the president sign into law that the only definition of Tea Bag is to dunk your nads in somebody's mouth."
>
> *Niko*
> *Tea Bag Now activist*
> *Madison, Wisconsin*

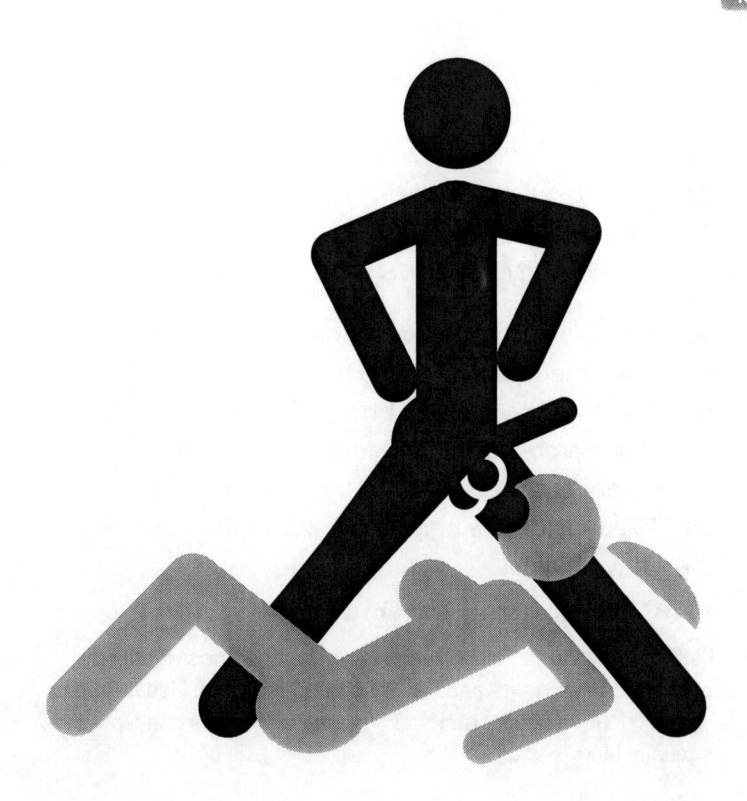

☐ Did It.

Date: ___/___/___   Partner: _____

My Personal
Enjoyment (1-10): ☐   My Partner's
Enjoyment (1-10): ☐

Comment: _____
_____
_____

TEA BAG

CHILI DOG
Mammae defaecatus conpressionis

To perform what's often described as "titty fucking on steroids," the man first defecates on his lover's chest. He then uses the slippery poo as lubricant to vigorously slide his member back and forth between her breasts, which serve as the "buns" to the "hotdog" and "poo-chili." A considerate partner allows his lover to lick off the "mayonnaise."

Props: Napkins, ketchup, mustard, red onions, sauerkraut (optional).

Hot Tip: Poo is an amazing natural lubricant composed entirely of organic ingredients and has no carbon footprint. Use it for all your lubrication needs: motor oil, masturbation, bike chain grease, squeaky hinges, etc.

Degree of Difficulty

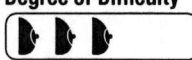

Degree of Nastiness

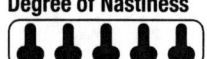

> "Seeing my husband's penis slide through his own poop on my chest was such a turn-on. I mean, here was a man who loved me enough to poop on me, fuck me in the poop and then cum on my face. It just makes you feel special."
>
> *Jeanie*
> *Waitress*
> *Vancouver, Canada*

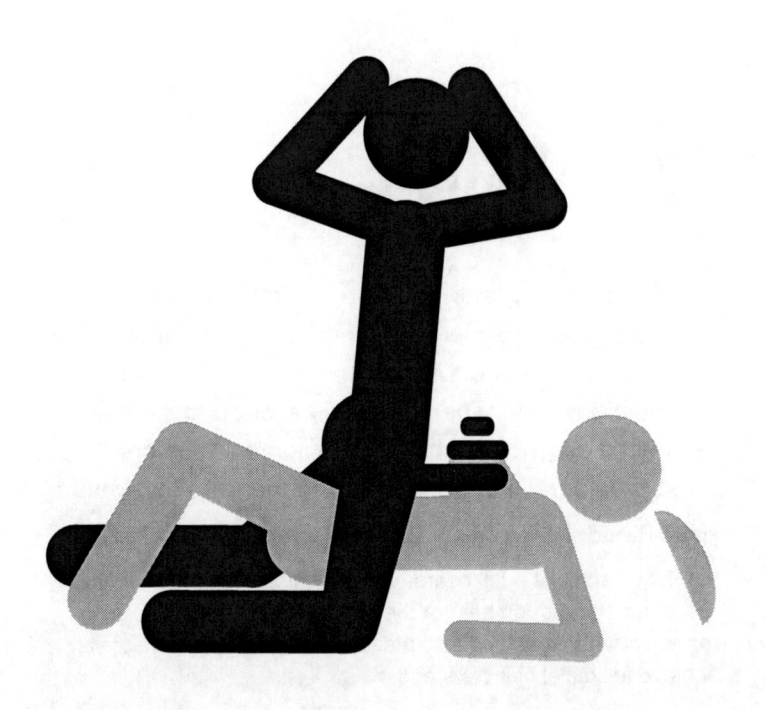

☐ Did It.

Date: ___/___/___ Partner: _____

My Personal
Enjoyment (1-10): ☐   My Partner's
Enjoyment (1-10): ☐

Comment: _____
_____
_____

CHILI DOG

ABE LINCOLN
Spermae barbatus

Half-fetish, half-prank, the Abe Lincoln involves ejaculating on a passed-out friend's face and then shaving one's own pubic hair to throw on the friend's unconscious face. The pubes will stick to the semen deposited around his chin and neck area, thus creating a most presidential of beards for the friend to awaken to.

Props: Razor, shaving cream, drunken friend, stove-pipe hat.

Hot Tip: To achieve a full beard, you may also have to shave your ass to gather enough hair for the task at hand. There's nothing more embarrassing (and less presidential) than being unable to achieve full facial hair coverage.

Degree of Difficulty

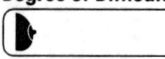

Degree of Nastiness

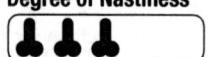

> *"I've always suffered from a crippling inability to grow facial hair, so my friends decided to surprise me by giving me an Abe Lincoln for my birthday. I felt like the luckiest boy in the whole world!"*
>
> Keith
> Acquisitions editor
> Berkeley, California

DIRTY SANCHEZ'S GUIDE TO BUCK NASTY SEX

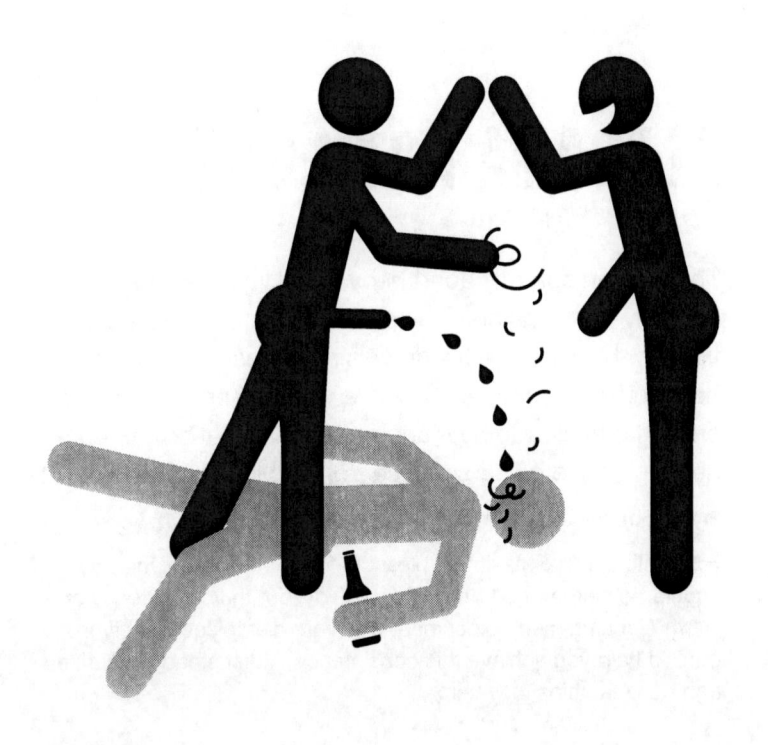

☐ Did It.

Date: ___/___/___   Partner: _____

My Personal
Enjoyment (1-10): ☐   My Partner's
Enjoyment (1-10): ☐

Comment: _____
_____
_____

ABE LINCOLN

ALABAMA HOT POCKET
Theca defaecatus

The woman spreads apart her vaginal lips while the man carefully positions his anus above her open crevice and fills it with shit. Once his bowels have been evacuated into her vagina, he proceeds to have vigorous sex with it and enjoy the explosive heat and gooeyness that erupts from her vagina like melted cheese from a blistering Hot Pocket.

Props: Speculum, poo funnel.

Hot Tip: To achieve maximum pleasure for both partners, the poo should be neither too firm nor too liquidy, but the consistency of warm Alabama mud. Experiment with your diet to see what types of food help you achieve this consistency. A diet steady in coffee and banana chips may help.

Degree of Difficulty

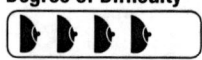

Degree of Nastiness

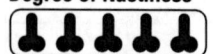

> "I love, love the Alabama Hot Pocket, but I wouldn't advise anybody to try it. You see, once you've had AHP, it's impossible to go back to regular sex. After my first Hot Pocket, my wife's vagina sans poop felt like the Sahara Desert."
>
> *Kevin*
> *Tech specialist*
> *Little Rock, Arkansas*

DIRTY SANCHEZ'S GUIDE TO BUCK NASTY SEX

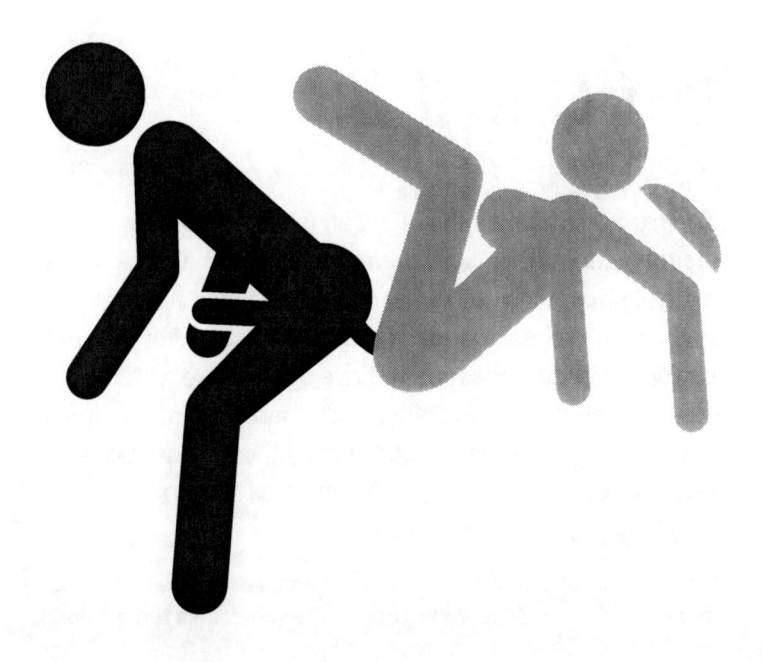

☐ **Did It.**

Date: ___/___/___ Partner: _____

My Personal
Enjoyment (1-10): ☐   My Partner's
Enjoyment (1-10): ☐

Comment: _____
_____
_____

ALABAMA HOT POCKET

HOT LUNCH
Cacatus manduco

The Hot Lunch takes the Hot Carl (see page 66) a steamy step further. One partner uses saran wrap to make a small pocket inside his/her mouth and then fills that pocket with feces (it doesn't matter whose). After this initial set-up, the man proceeds to have intercourse with the poo pocket, breaking through the saran wrap at the final, climatic second to fill his lover's mouth with a delicious fusion of cum and dump, also known as "cump."

Props: Saran wrap.

Hot Tip: "Cump" is a dish best served warm, so be sure to use the freshest feces available and to not let the intercourse run overlong, lest the poop begin to cool and solidify.

Degree of Difficulty

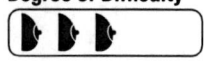

Degree of Nastiness

> "The sexual pleasure of the Hot Lunch speaks for itself, but less obvious is the way in which it has helped millions of people overcome their aversions to actual hot lunches by replacing terrifying memories of sweaty school cafeteria food with beautiful, aromatic mouthfuls of cump."
>
> *Ricardo*
> *Cump lobbyist*
> *Washington, D.C.*

DIRTY SANCHEZ'S GUIDE TO BUCK NASTY SEX

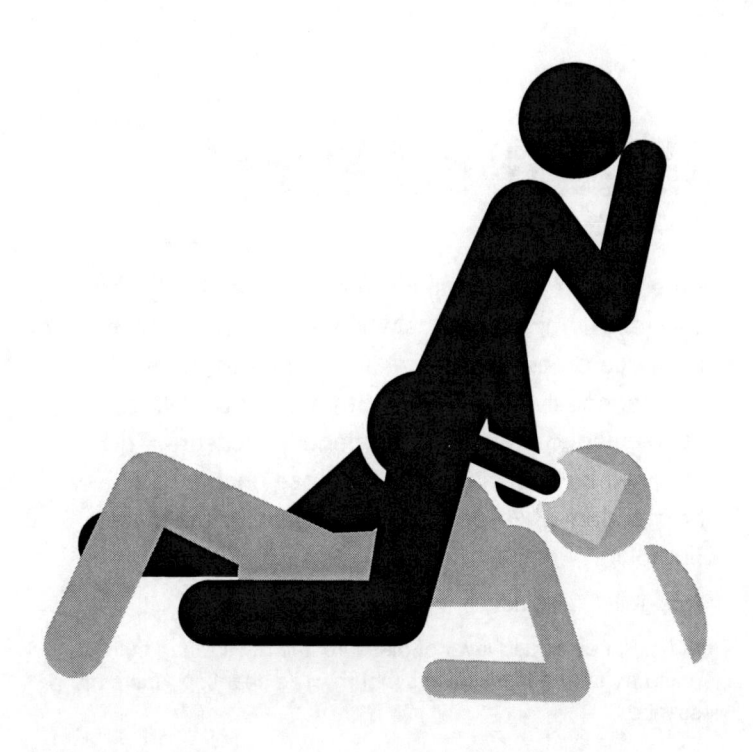

☐ Did It.

Date: ___/___/___ Partner: _____

My Personal Enjoyment (1-10): ☐   My Partner's Enjoyment (1-10): ☐

Comment: _____
_____
_____

HOT LUNCH

REVERSE BLUMPKIN
Analingus miatus

A member of the Blumpkin (see page 74) family, the Reverse Blumpkin occurs when a woman performs analingus on her partner while he urinates, thus simultaneously stimulating both anus and urethra in a two-headed monster of erogenous pleasure. This fetish works especially well for those unable to achieve the erection-while-pooping necessary for the classic Blumpkin.

Props: Toilet, full bladder.

Hot Tip: For an added layer of pleasure, the micturating man should try farting in his lover's mouth while chanting "Taste my essence."

Degree of Difficulty

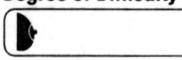

Degree of Nastiness

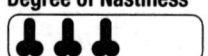

> *"For those of us who are sexually disabled, the Reverse Blumpkin is a godsend. Though I can't achieve an erection, I can piss and get my butthole eaten out like there's no tomorrow."*
>
> Todd
> Truck driver
> Fresno, California

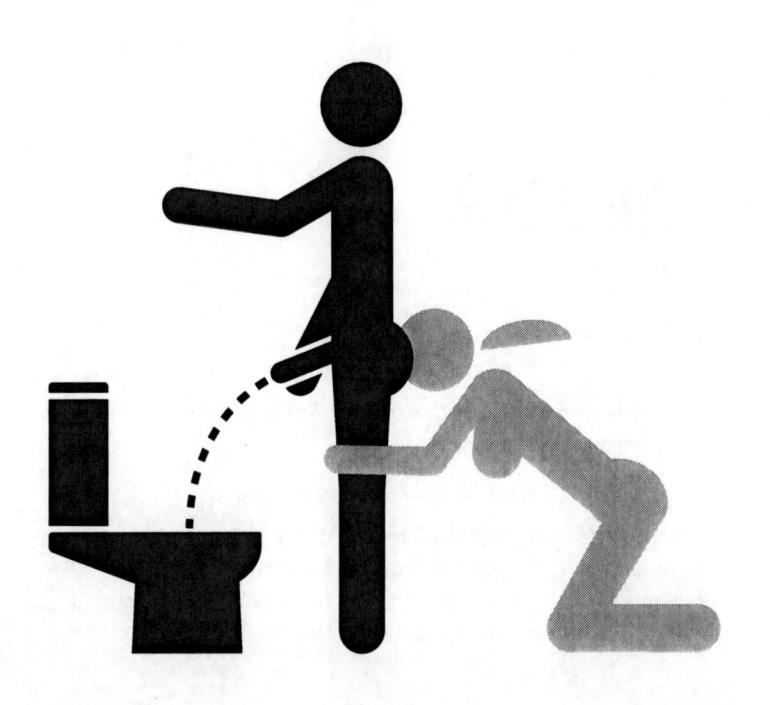

☐ Did It.

Date: ___/___/___   Partner: _____

My Personal Enjoyment (1-10): ☐   My Partner's Enjoyment (1-10): ☐

Comment: _____
_____
_____

REVERSE BLUMPKIN

PINK SOCK
Colus impilium

During a rigorous session of anal intercourse, the man thrusts so vigorously that his partner's lower intestine is actually pulled out of the anus to dangle from the rectum like a crimson stocking.

Props: Emergency Medical Services, anal surgeon.

Hot Tip: To effectively pull the intestine out of the anus, the intestinal wall must catch on the rim of the penis. So be sure to use as little lubrication as possible and simply jam the penis roughly into the buttocks. Continue to thrust until you "get a bite."

Degree of Difficulty

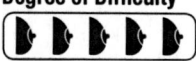

Degree of Nastiness

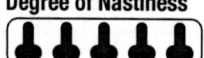

> "I wouldn't say that I regret my many Pink Sockings, since they are, obviously, enormously pleasurable, but they have made it difficult for my sphincter to hold back the tides, so to speak."
>
> *Anna*
> *Vintner*
> *Sonoma, California*

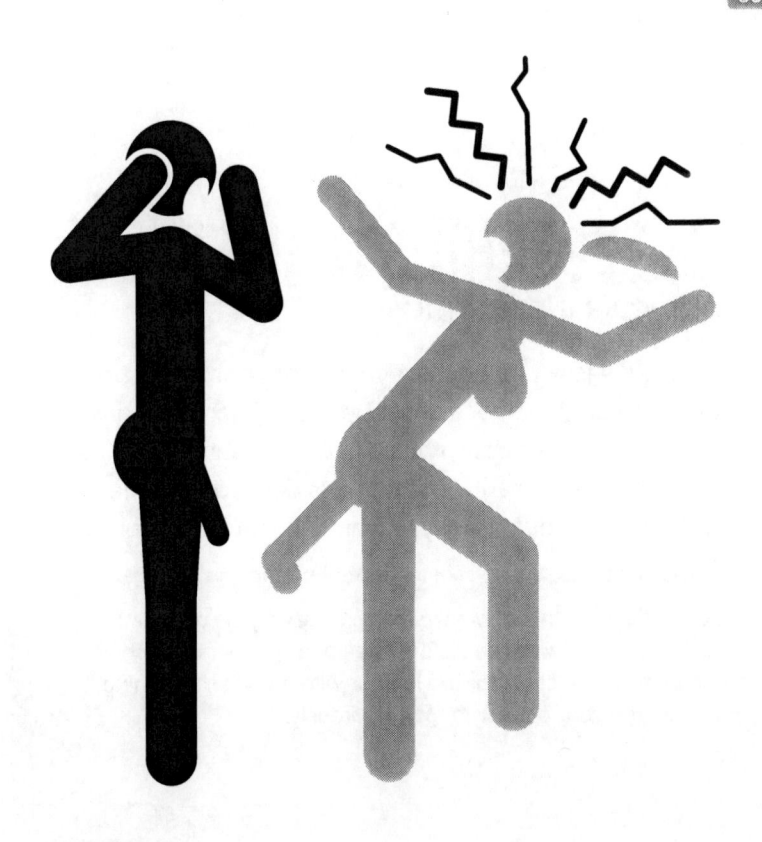

☐ **Did It.**

Date: ___/___/___   Partner: _____

My Personal
Enjoyment (1-10): ☐   My Partner's
Enjoyment (1-10): ☐

Comment: _____
_____
_____

PINK SOCK

CLEVELAND STEAMER
Navicula clevelandus

During a session of coitus, either partner proceeds to defecate on the other's chest before rocking back and forth across the malodorous pile like a steamroller moving over soft, loamy earth. The name is derived from the Midwestern industrial city in which the fetish was born.

Props: Laxatives, broad-chested sexual partner.

Hot Tip: Feces — though warm when first leaving the body — cools quite rapidly, and can cause the "steamed" partner to catch cold if it's left on the chest for too long or with too little "steaming." Encourage your partner to rock vigorously.

Degree of Difficulty

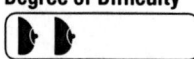

Degree of Nastiness

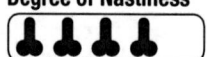

> *"Like New York–style pizza, a Cleveland Steamer is great anywhere, but it's always best at the source. They made it famous for a reason, ya know?"*
>
> Henry
> Commercial pilot
> Newark, New Jersey

DIRTY SANCHEZ'S GUIDE TO BUCK NASTY SEX

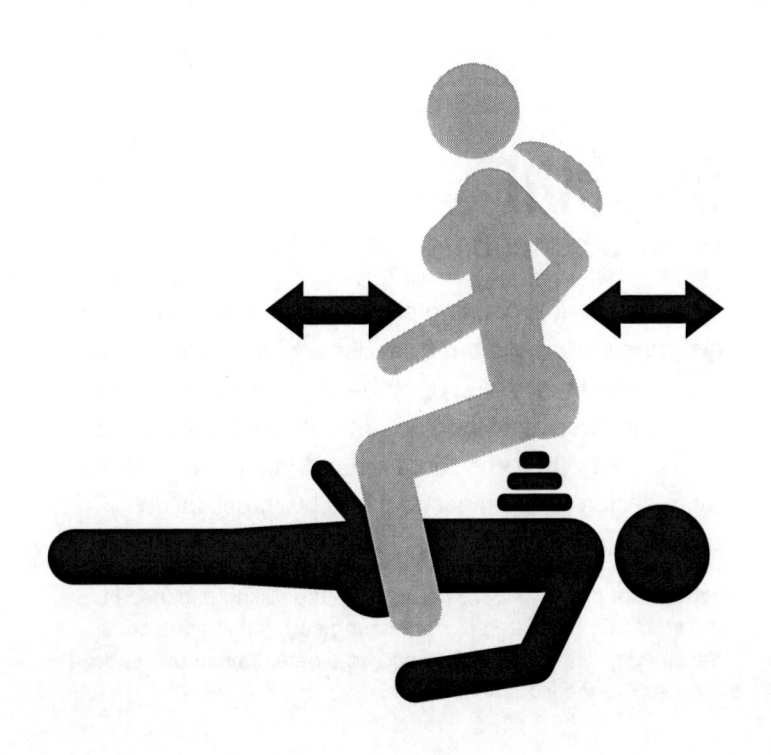

☐ Did It.

Date: ___/___/___   Partner: _____

My Personal Enjoyment (1-10): ☐   My Partner's Enjoyment (1-10): ☐

Comment: _____
_____
_____

CLEVELAND STEAMER

HOUDINI
Fellacio concubitis

As a man is approaching climax while rear-entering his partner, he pulls out from her vaginal embrace and expectorates, or spits, upon her back, thus deceiving her — like a sexual Houdini — into thinking that he has ejaculated. When she turns around, he reveals the truth by releasing his seminal fluid into her face. Ta-da!

Props: Invisible handcuffs, magic saw, rabbit, hat.

Hot Tip: Houdini died while performing after being punched in the stomach. It's therefore not recommended that you combine the Houdini with more violent acts to create dangerous hybrid fetishes like the Houdonki Punch.

Degree of Difficulty

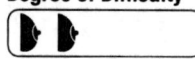

Degree of Nastiness

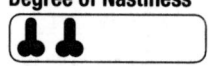

> "She who fakes orgasm will be Houdinied in return."
> *Ancient Chinese proverb*

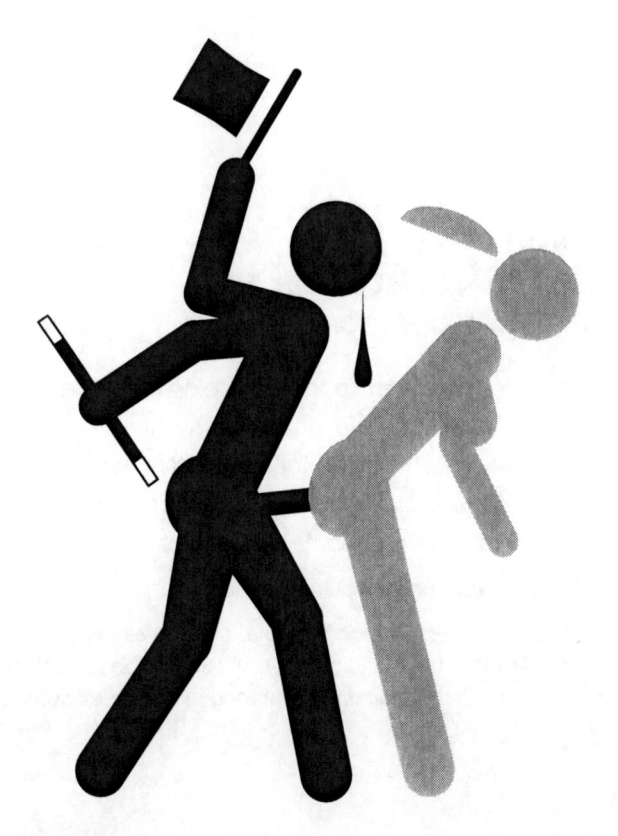

☐ Did It.

Date: ___/___/___   Partner: _____

My Personal Enjoyment (1-10): ☐   My Partner's Enjoyment (1-10): ☐

Comment: _____
_____
_____

HOUDINI

CUNNILUMPKIN
Cunnilingus defaecatus

The female counterpart to the Blumpkin (see page 74), the Cunnilumpkin is a two-part fetish. While the woman is being sexed orally on the toilet, she discharges her excrement, thus allowing her to experience the twin pleasures of sexual and scatological ecstasy.

Props: Customized Cunnilumpkin toilet seat.

Hot Tip: Unless one enjoys coprophagia, or poop eating, it is recommended that the man limit his oral explorations strictly to the clitoral area to avoid the possibility of tongue and feces contact.

Degree of Difficulty

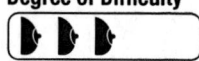

Degree of Nastiness

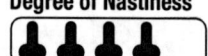

> "Many men fear Cunnilumpkin because of an internalized phobia of the oft-mythologized anu detanta, or fanged anus."
>
> Sue
> Sexual theorist
> Palo Alto, California

☐ Did It.

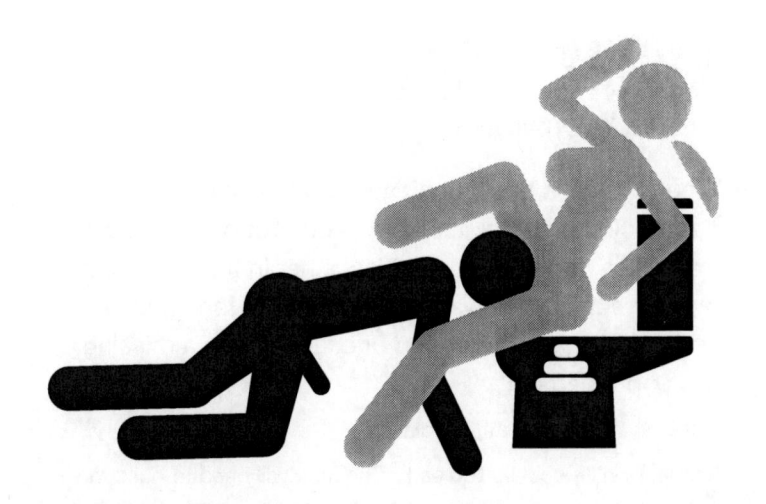

Date: ___/___/___   Partner: _____

My Personal
Enjoyment (1-10): ☐   My Partner's
Enjoyment (1-10): ☐

Comment: _____
_____
_____

CUNNILUMPKIN

ANGRY PIRATE
Pirata iracundia

When a man is orally copulating with a woman, just before climax, he pulls his member out of her mouth, ejaculates into her eye, and kicks her in the shin. This twin assault causes his female partner to rant, squint and hobble like an enraged buccaneer with a missing eye and a peg leg.

Props: Steel-toed boots, spyglass.

Hot Tip: Don't ejaculate too early. The man will need to build the projectile force of his semen in order to deposit it cleanly into the female's eye, rather than allowing it to dribble slowly over the glans, or head, of the penis.

Degree of Difficulty

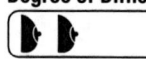

Degree of Nastiness

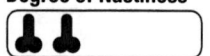

> "Back in the '80s, everybody was Angry Pirating each other left and right. But then, everybody got scared of eye herpes and you couldn't pay to Angry Pirate. Or when you did, you had to wear glasses. But who wants to do that? Angry Pirating with glasses is like showering with your socks on."
>
> *Marcus*
> *Coffee shop owner*
> *San Francisco, California*

DIRTY SANCHEZ'S GUIDE TO BUCK NASTY SEX

☐ Did It.

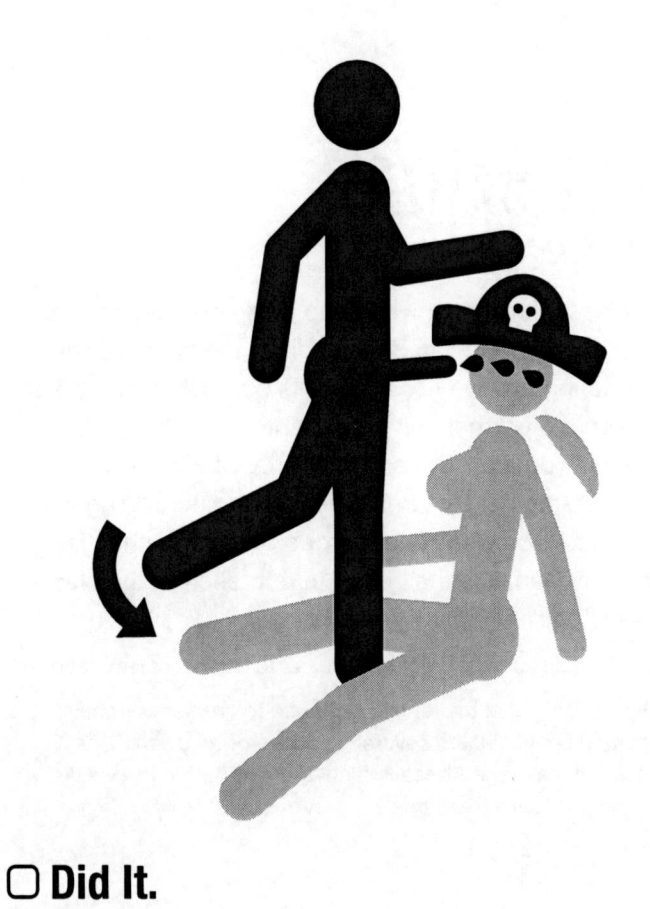

Date: ___/___/___   Partner: _____

My Personal
Enjoyment (1-10): ☐   My Partner's
Enjoyment (1-10): ☐

Comment: _____
_____
_____

ANGRY PIRATE

TONY DANZA
Verpae percisis

This classic fetish involves deep rear-entry penetration and rhythmic pounding on the part of the male. At any point during his exertions, he yells out "Who's the boss?" to which his partner will predictably, if confusedly, respond "You are!" But she is wrong, of course, and the male corrects her by turning her around, stropping her across the face with his engorged penis and chastising, "No, Tony Danza is the boss!" in reference to the classic family sitcom.

Props: Old episodes of *Who's the Boss?* for further re-education

Hot Tip: To fairly give the female a chance to answer correctly, the couple should watch several episodes of *Who's the Boss?* and take at least one Alyssa Milano–themed quiz in the weeks preceding sexual intercourse.

Degree of Difficulty

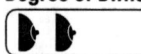

Degree of Nastiness

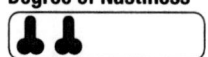

> *"Honestly, anybody who doesn't know that Tony Danza is the boss deserves to take a cock across the face."*
>
> Peggy
> Accountant
> New Haven, Connecticut

DIRTY SANCHEZ'S GUIDE TO BUCK NASTY SEX

Who's the BOSS?

Tony Danza!

Tony Danza!

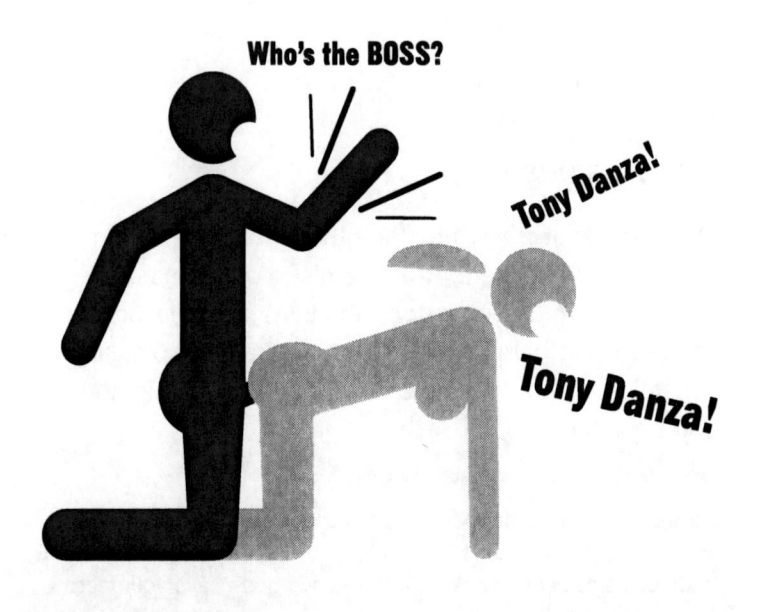

☐ Did It.

Date: ___/___/___　Partner: _____

My Personal Enjoyment (1-10): ☐　My Partner's Enjoyment (1-10): ☐

Comment: _____
_____
_____

TONY DANZA

HOT CARL
Carlotus aestuo

One partner gently wraps the other's face with saran wrap (leaving space for the nostrils to breathe) before proceeding to defecate upon the thin, taught layer of plastic. The other partner experiences a most pleasing sensation as warm excreta is deposited upon his/her countenance.

Props: Saran wrap, moist towelettes.

Hot Tip: Summoning poop at will is hard work. If you're planning to surprise your lover with a Hot Carl later in the evening, be sure not to defecate earlier in the day. As the saying goes, save your feces for the ones you love.

Degree of Difficulty

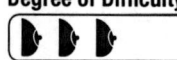

Degree of Nastiness

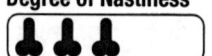

> "Like with most couples, the magic of having my husband take a dump on my face started to fade after a few years. But bringing saran wrap into the equation really helped to spice things up."
>
> Sally
> Housewife
> Omaha, Nebraska

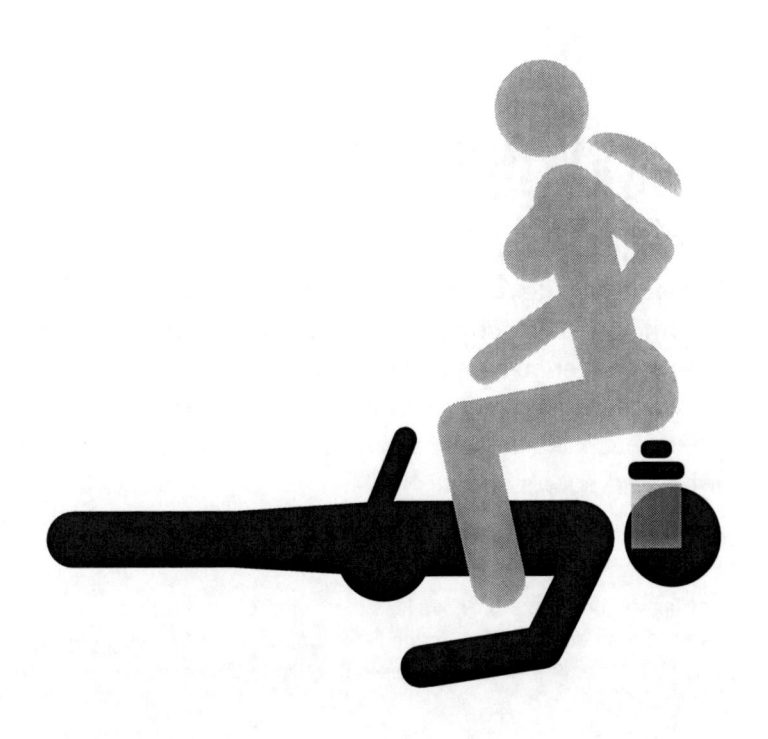

☐ Did It.

Date: ___/___/___   Partner: _____

My Personal Enjoyment (1-10): ☐   My Partner's Enjoyment (1-10): ☐

Comment: _____
_____
_____

HOT CARL

ANGRY DRAGON
Irascor draconis

Immediately after the man ejaculates into his partner's mouth during oral copulation, he delivers a jarring blow to the rear of her cranium, thus forcing his shocked partner to suddenly gasp and expunge his semen through her nose, much like the wisps of smoke that trickle from an irritated dragon's snout.

Props: Tissue, ice (for jarring hand), pro-dragon literature to demonstrate coolness of dragons.

Hot Tip: Women tend to derive less pleasure from the Angry Dragon than do men. But, much like dragons, women love jewels, and have been known to be more receptive to this fetish when proffered with gold.

Degree of Difficulty

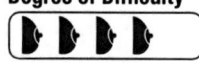

Degree of Nastiness

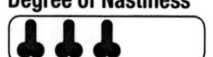

"My students just weren't understanding how real the threat of dragons was to medieval peasants. But after I demonstrated the Angry Dragon for them, it all just clicked."

Peter
10th-grade history teacher
Des Moines, Iowa

Thump!

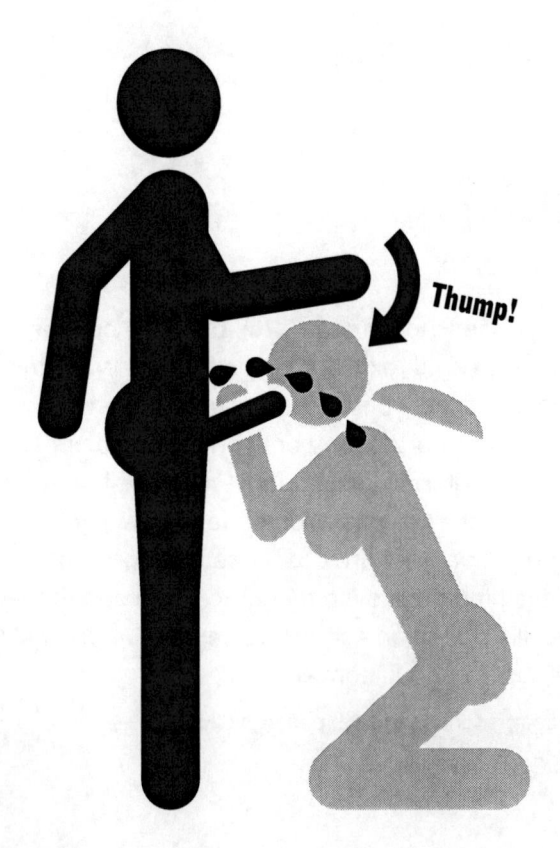

☐ Did It.

Date: ___/___/___ Partner: _____

My Personal
Enjoyment (1-10): ☐

My Partner's
Enjoyment (1-10): ☐

Comment: _____
_____
_____

ANGRY DRAGON

BRONCO
Equus ferus

Similar to the Rodeo (page 126), but sans crowds, the Bronco is a quick, exhilarating ride for either partner. Mid-coitus, simply begin screaming out the wrong name for your partner and hold on as long as possible. Most men prefer an initial doggy-style position, with a firm grip on the breasts. Women tend to enjoy the swift, bucking action from on top. Remember, once it's over, the explaining begins, so try not to use a common name (especially one of an acquaintance) and be prepared for a potentially serious conversation.

Props: Leather chaps, bullwhip, first-aid kit.

Hot Tip: Gird your loins.

Degree of Difficulty

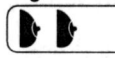

Degree of Nastiness

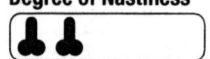

> *"Thanks to this classy little move, I am now divorced. Apparently I forgot the name of my wife's pretty younger sister. Midway through the Bronco, I remembered it."*
>
> *George*
> *Unemployed*
> *El Paso, Texas*

DIRTY SANCHEZ'S GUIDE TO BUCK NASTY SEX

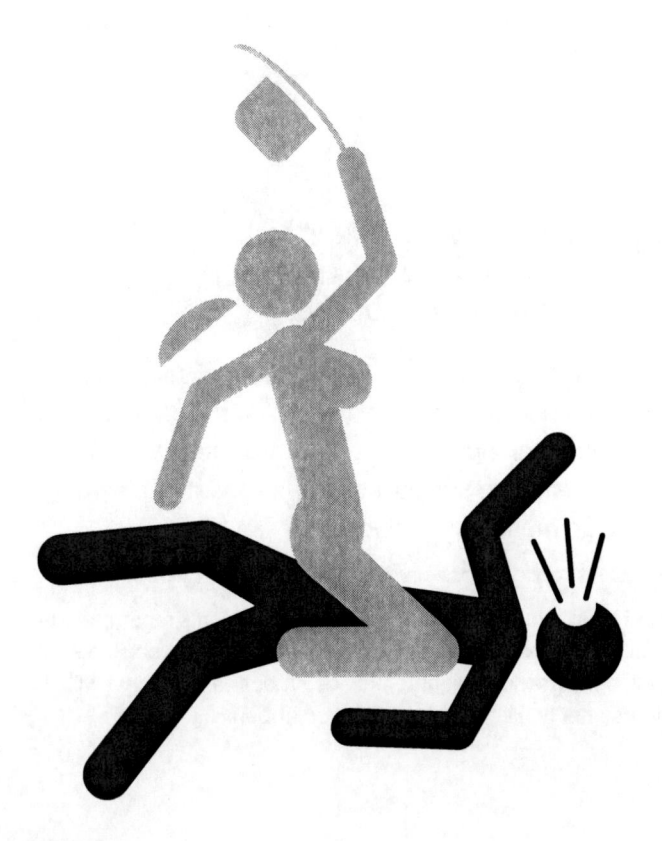

☐ Did It.

Date: ___/___/___ Partner: _____

My Personal
Enjoyment (1-10): ☐

My Partner's
Enjoyment (1-10): ☐

Comment: _____
_____
_____

BRONCO

DIRTY SANCHEZ
Clunis concubitis barba

After a man and woman engage in anal sex, the male removes his still-erect member from his partner's rectum and rubs it along her upper lip, thus creating a sort of fecal mustachio supposedly reminiscent of a scraggly Mexican mustache, or *bigote*.

Props: Astroglide, nose plugs, mustache tracing kit.

Hot Tip: To avoid a patchy, broken mustache, it's recommended that the woman ingest an oily, difficult-to-digest cuisine such as Indian the previous night to provide smooth excreta that will glide across her lip like a high-end ballpoint pen.

Degree of Difficulty

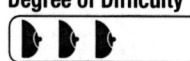

Degree of Nastiness

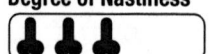

> "Women love being Dirty Sanchezed because of the power reversal and gender switch that comes from having a typically masculine mustache painted across their face with a penis."
>
> *Anita*
> *Sexual psychologist*
> *Fresno, California*

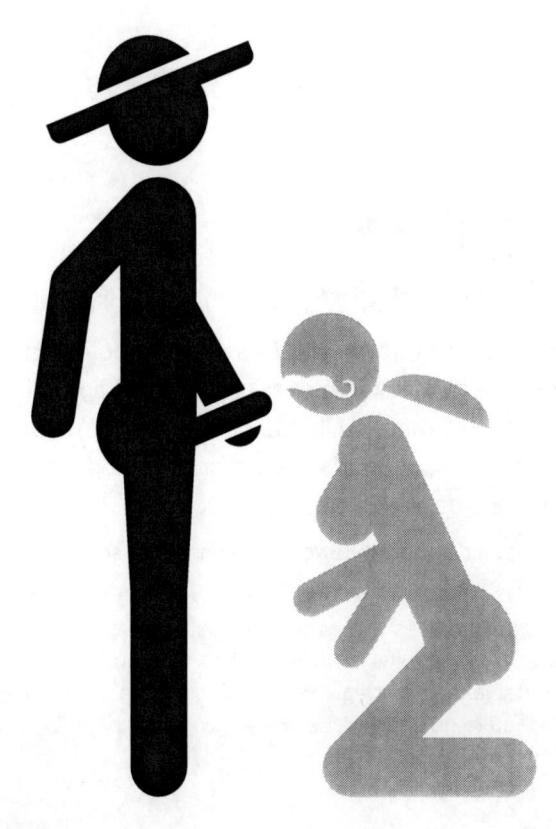

☐ Did It.

Date: ___/___/___   Partner: _____

My Personal Enjoyment (1-10): ☐   My Partner's Enjoyment (1-10): ☐

Comment: _____
_____
_____

DIRTY SANCHEZ

BLUMPKIN
Fellatio defecatus

It's a race to the throne with this exciting but simple sex act. The man takes a seat on the toilet and begins his bowel movement while his partner performs oral sex during defecation. If timed properly, the first scat should coincide with a potent orgasm.

Props: Knee pads or plush towel, air freshener or scented candle. plumbing.

Hot Tip: When it comes to a good Blumpkin, the key is fiber, fiber, fiber. Nothing ruins more Blumpkins worldwide than the uncomfortable bout of irregularity or constipation. Know when and how you're going to go before enticing your partner.

Degree of Difficulty

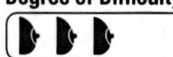

Degree of Nastiness

> *"Once you get over the smell, the act is very pleasureful. Henry always finishes the paper at the same time. Then just hop in the shower for round two!"*
>
> Michelle
> *Dermatologist*
> *St. Cloud, Minnesota*

DIRTY SANCHEZ'S GUIDE TO BUCK NASTY SEX

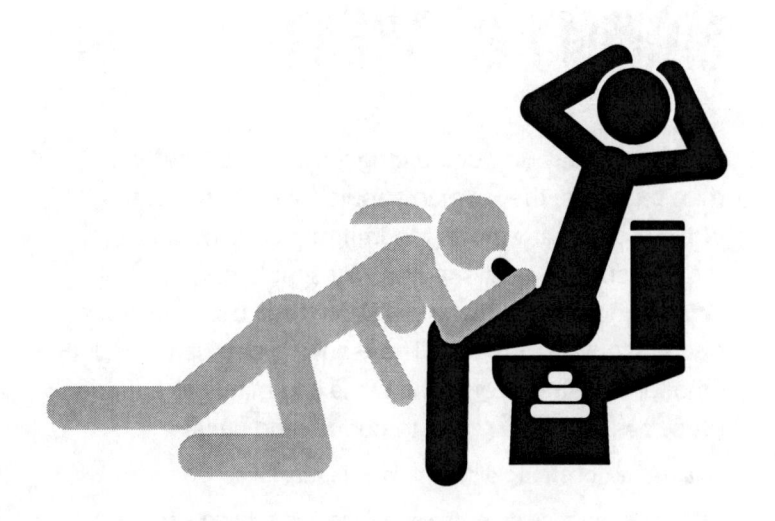

☐ Did It.

Date: ___/___/___   Partner: _____

My Personal Enjoyment (1-10): ☐   My Partner's Enjoyment (1-10): ☐

Comment: _____
_____
_____

BLUMPKIN

MOMMY DEAREST
Mater amor

A little role playing goes a long way. Just before the man orgasms, the woman should take on the role of his mother, attempting to imitate her voice and mannerisms as best she can. Try simple phrases like "Who's mommy's little angel?" or "Shh, don't tell your daddy I let you stay up." The resulting confusion and emotional distress turns the climaxing man into a tender prepubescent boy, ready to cuddle and suckle.

Props: A mix of strong discipline and tender love.

Hot Tip: Always include a little spanking and schedule an appointment for couple's therapy before attempting a Mommy Dearest.

Degree of Difficulty

Degree of Nastiness

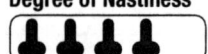

"Nothing arouses the man like the Oedipus complex and touching his penis at the same time. Ladies, if you want a man to fall in love with you, this is the secret. It just works."

Abby
Clinical psychologist
Atlanta, Georgia

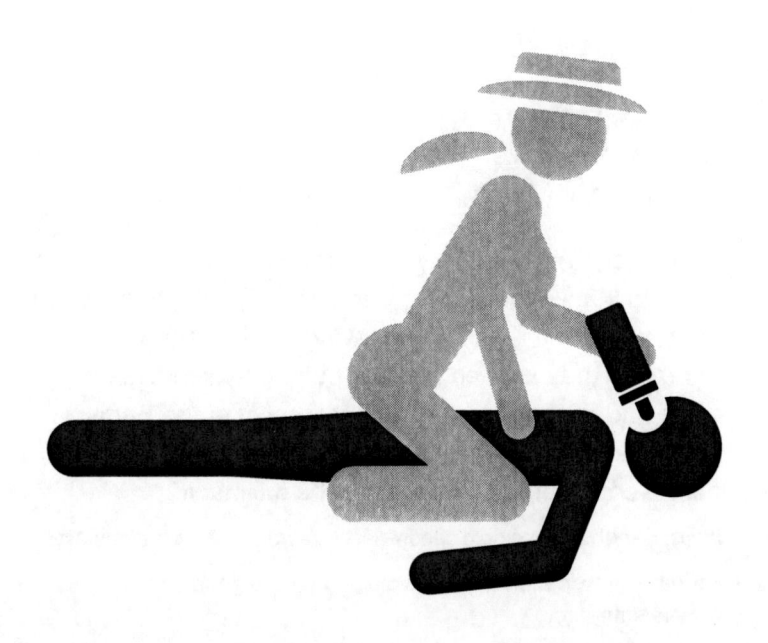

☐ Did It.

Date: ___/___/___   Partner: _____

My Personal
Enjoyment (1-10): ☐   My Partner's
Enjoyment (1-10): ☐

Comment: _____
_____
_____

MOMMY DEAREST

BURNING MAN
Sordesco

Otherwise known simply as "Dirty Hippy Sex," Burning Man involves both partners forgetting to shower for at least four days before having sex in a sandbox. For most, the experience takes putting hygienic ideals aside and giving in to the spiritual power of the Earth. Try taking some drugs and setting something on fire before copulating to experience the full magic.

Props: Sandbox/litter box/beach/desert, acid/mushrooms/ecstasy.

Hot Tip: Throw in a bit of chlamydia and you've got a sexual double entendre.

Degree of Difficulty

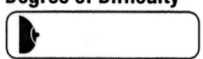

Degree of Nastiness

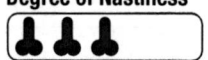

> "It's totally the best way to make love, man. It's like Adam and Eve in the garden, just naked and free."
>
> *Rainbow Starship*
> *Healer*
> *Bangor, Maine*

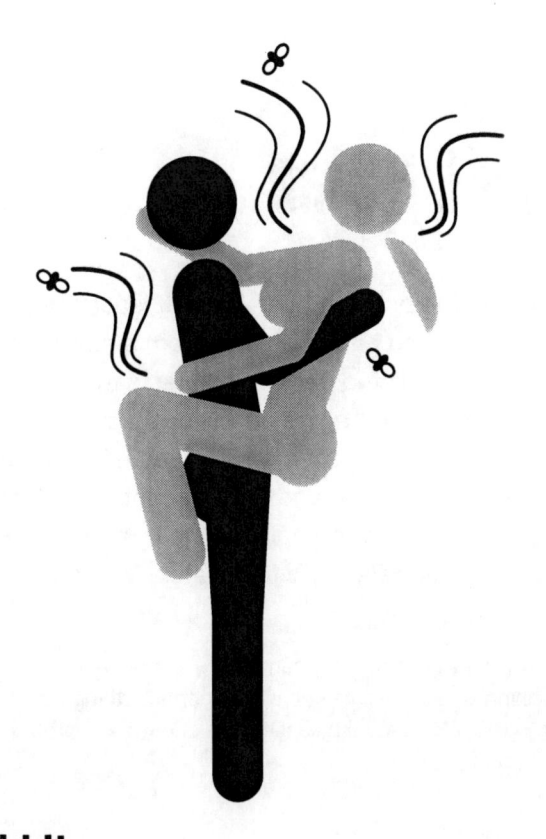

☐ Did It.

Date: ___/___/___   Partner: _____

My Personal Enjoyment (1-10): ☐   My Partner's Enjoyment (1-10): ☐

Comment: _____
_____
_____

BURNING MAN

CAMEL HUMP
Aqua camelus

The Camel Hump works best when at least one partner is cotton-mouthed and hung over from a night out on the town. The afflicted partner initiates a morning session with the other, then begins obnoxiously spitting in the lover's face. The pungent morning breath imbues the sticky saliva with a wild and exotic scent. If the gob catcher comments or complains, the partner simply gets up and wanders off to find water.

Props: A sour disposition.

Hot Tip: If you haven't heard a camel sing, it's quite beautiful. Try moaning a sound somewhere between a birthing cow and a dying cat — it's a crowd pleaser and a sure way to arouse the neighbors.

Degree of Difficulty

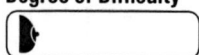

Degree of Nastiness

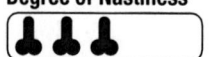

> "The whole 'hair of the dog' thing never helped me get over a hangover. But 'morning at the zoo' always seems to do the trick."
>
> Jack
> Bartender
> Boston, Massachusetts

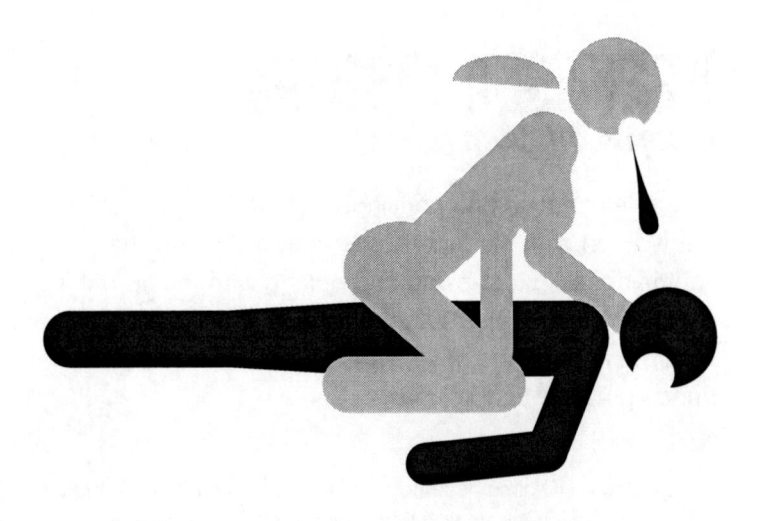

☐ Did It.

Date: ___/___/___   Partner: _____

My Personal Enjoyment (1-10): ☐   My Partner's Enjoyment (1-10): ☐

Comment: _____
_____
_____

CAMEL HUMP

DEEP-SEA FISHING
Odorus officium

A simple variation on cunnilingus: instead of pleasuring the woman with his mouth, the man dives into the vagina nose-first, stroking and poking with the tip of his protuberance. Firmer than the tongue and more sensitive than the fingers, the nose is the perfect instrument for bringing a woman to climax.

Props: Saline nasal spray, nose plug.

Hot Tip: Under NO circumstances should the man breathe through his nose while "in the drink." Take deep, methodical breaths through an open mouth.

Degree of Difficulty

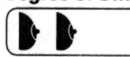

Degree of Nastiness

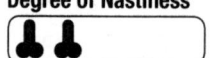

"I'm a lawyer, and I need my tongue rested to do business, so oral sex for my wife is out of the question. If she wants pleasure, she has three options: fingers, nose, dick. She says she likes the biggest, so that's what I give her."

Richard
Corporate attorney
Los Angeles, California

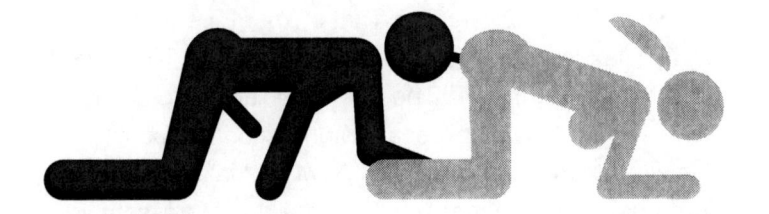

☐ Did It.

Date: ___/___/___   Partner: _____

My Personal
Enjoyment (1-10): ☐
My Partner's
Enjoyment (1-10): ☐

Comment: _____
_____
_____

DEEP-SEA FISHING

HIGHBALL
Fumo magus

Known in Britain as the "Put That in Your Pipe and Smoke It," this sexual ending is perfect for those who like to finish up with a little puff-puff. The man ejaculates into a waiting water bong, allowing his seed to drip into the water. The woman then packs a fresh bowl and takes a long, sumptuous hit. The marijuana, normally a depressant, is turned into a powerful aphrodisiac for both partners.

Props: Quality marijuana strain, glass bong, food.

Hot Tip: Try filling the bong with ice before use. As the hot sperm slips and slides down the cubes, both the water and seed will cool and congeal, creating a natural filter for the smoke, resulting in cool, salty hits.

Degree of Difficulty

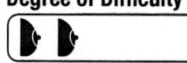

Degree of Nastiness

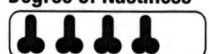

> *"I hate how harsh smoke can be, even out of a bong. For some reason, Steve's come just smoothes everything out. It's crazy. It tastes like strawberries!"*
>
> Hannah
> Student
> San Diego, California

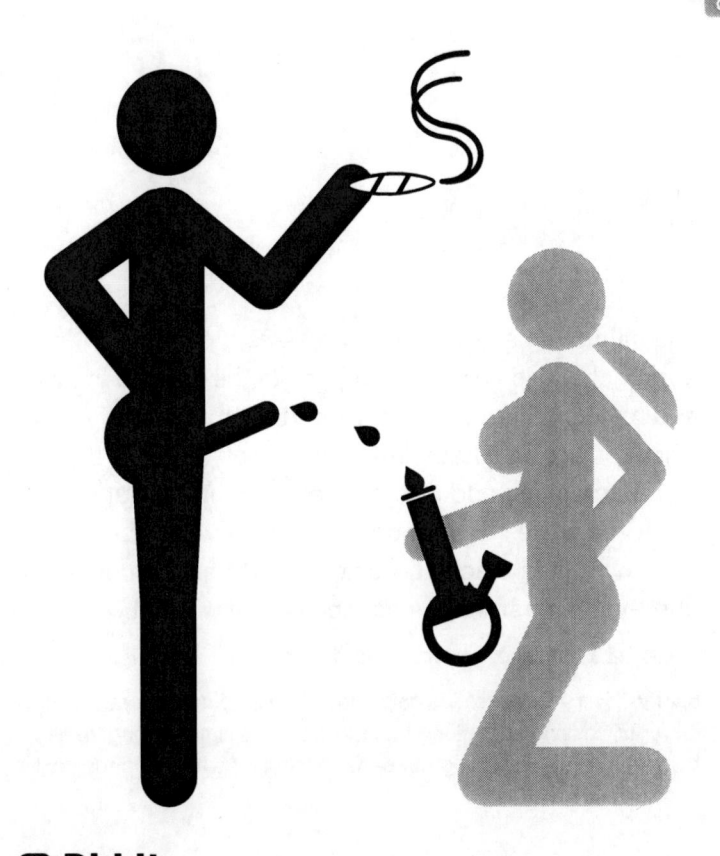

☐ Did It.

Date: ___/___/___   Partner: _____

My Personal
Enjoyment (1-10): ☐   My Partner's
Enjoyment (1-10): ☐

Comment: _____
_____
_____

HIGHBALL

KAMIKAZE
Prolixus neco

The ultimate male-fantasy finale—as the man approaches his finish in doggy-style, he yells "banzai!" and makes a hard dive for his partner's puckered anus. Chances are he'll never make the small target at such a speed, crashing and burning before contact. But every once in a while . . . kaboom! No matter what, the man ends up a little black and blue, but when it comes to the one-eyed emperor, the sacrifice is well worth it.

Props: Glass of sake, samurai sword, good aim.

Hot Tip: Diversionary tactics help a lot when it comes to a successful entry. Try tossing something into the woman's sightline or give her hair a gentle tug, anything to keep her mind off what happens next.

Degree of Difficulty

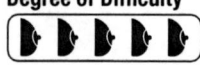

Degree of Nastiness

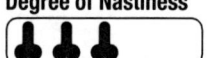

> *"I absolutely hate it when my boyfriend Kamikazes me. So I started wearing high heels during sex. Now when he makes a move for my ass hole, he gets a stiletto in his. Payback's a bitch."*
>
> *Carrie*
> *Fashion consultant*
> *Jersey City, New Jersey*

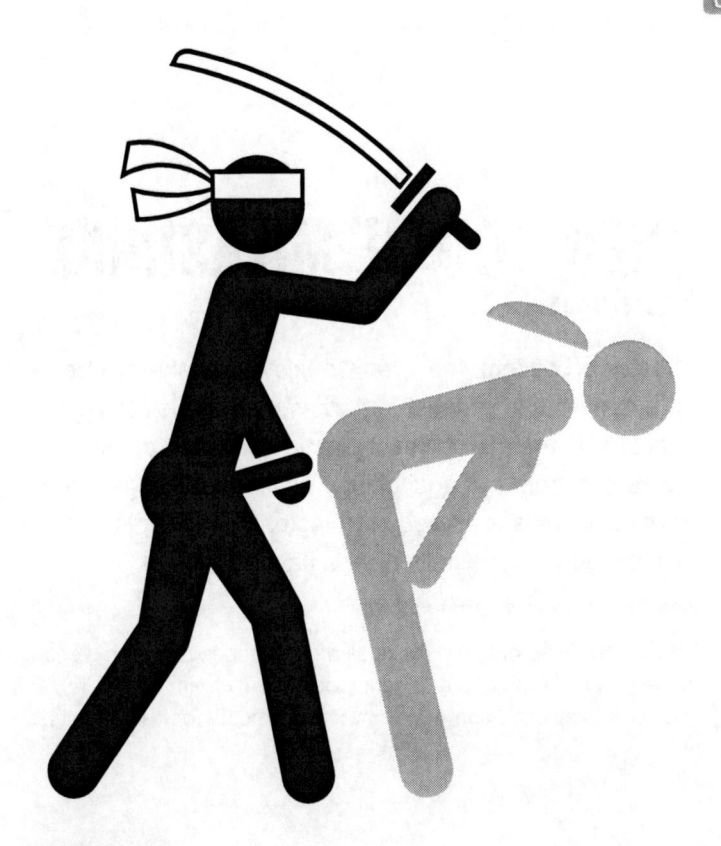

☐ Did It.

Date: ___/___/___   Partner: _____

My Personal Enjoyment (1-10): ☐   My Partner's Enjoyment (1-10): ☐

Comment: _____
_____
_____

KAMIKAZE

OREO COOKIE MILKSHAKE
Lac fimus

A fast-food delight, the Oreo Cookie Milkshake is a treat for him alone. After finishing up with an arousing session of anal sex, the man takes a plastic straw and sucks out the semen from her anal cavity. While the strange, tangy mixture of fluids is an acquired taste, most people find it very pleasing, especially after a flavorful dinner.

Props: Plastic straw, strong stomach.

Hot Tip: What she eats will make all the difference between a shake made of real Oreos and a generic cookies 'n' cream rip off. Try fiber-rich foods and some well-marinated meats for best results.

Degree of Difficulty

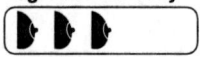

Degree of Nastiness

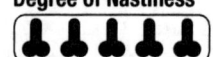

> "I used to get the milkshakes at fast-food restaurants, but they're so damn expensive. Making them at home is just as easy and a whole lot more fun!"
>
> *Nick*
> *Coffee shop owner*
> *Hannibal, Missouri*

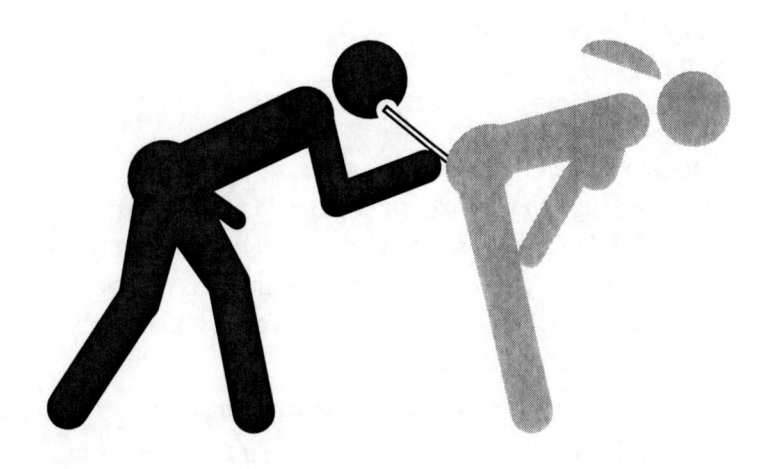

☐ Did It.

Date: ___/___/___   Partner: _____

My Personal Enjoyment (1-10): ☐   My Partner's Enjoyment (1-10): ☐

Comment: _____
_____
_____

OREO COOKIE MILKSHAKE

PREDATOR
Fimus faeces

After sex, when the woman goes to the bathroom to clean up, the man should defecate in his hands and smear the feces on his face and body. Not only terrifying and disturbing to those who may venture into the room, this simple move is a great way to cover up the body's heat signature.

Props: Air-cooled Gatling gun, counter-weighted trap.

Hot Tip: While many people say it's the face and arms that matter, don't be fooled into half-assing a Predator—make sure your entire body is covered. The most heat emanating from your body at this moment will be your groin, so cover up and keep moving.

Degree of Difficulty

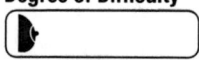

Degree of Nastiness

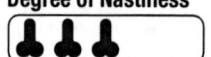

> "Nothing'll make you more of a sexual Tyrannosaurus than pulling this on your girl. She'll freak, she'll squeal, she'll feel like she's back in the fucking jungle."
>
> *Buck*
> *Insurance agent*
> *Salt Lake City, Utah*

DIRTY SANCHEZ'S GUIDE TO BUCK NASTY SEX

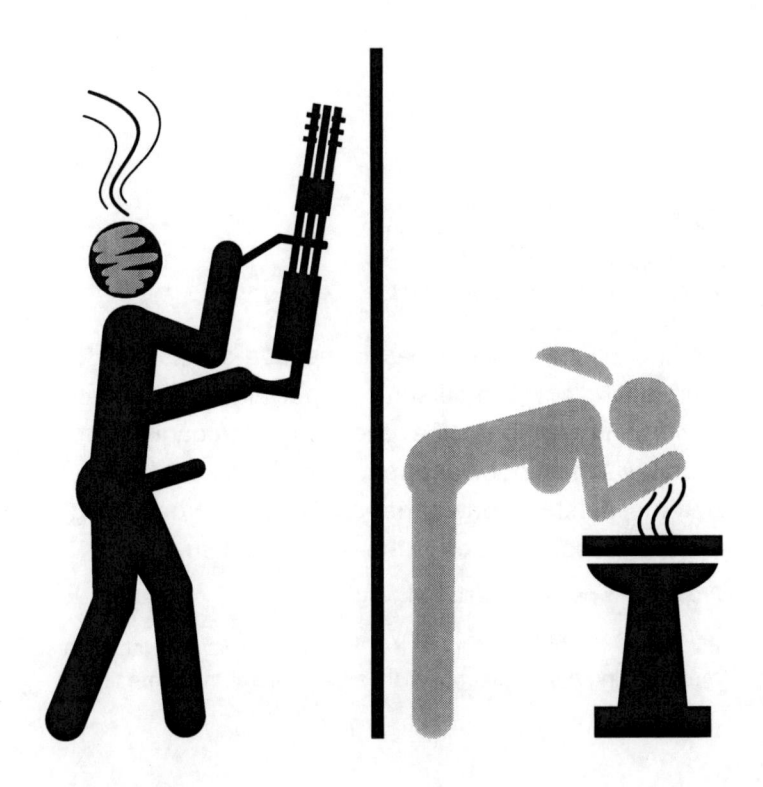

☐ Did It.

Date: ___/___/___ Partner: _____

My Personal
Enjoyment (1-10): ☐   My Partner's
Enjoyment (1-10): ☐

Comment: _____
_____
_____

PREDATOR

PTERODACTYL
Pennipotenti antiquus

Adding a third man to a classic ménage-a-trois can be intimidating and cumbersome, especially when it comes to finishing everyone off at once. The Pterodactyl is one of today's most popular approaches. The woman, on her knees, felates one of her partners while delivering simultaneous handjobs to the other two men.

Props: Knee pads, lube, paleontologist.

Hot Tip: Try finishing up with a "K-T Boundary *bukake*," with all three men sending their meteoric finishes faceward at the same time.

Degree of Difficulty

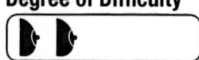

Degree of Nastiness

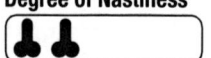

> "Obviously, group sex is kind of my thing, and nothing looks better on camera than finishing off three cocks at the same time. It's all about rhythm and keeping everything in synch."
>
> *Bambi Hotlips*
> Porn star
> Bakersfield, California

DIRTY SANCHEZ'S GUIDE TO BUCK NASTY SEX

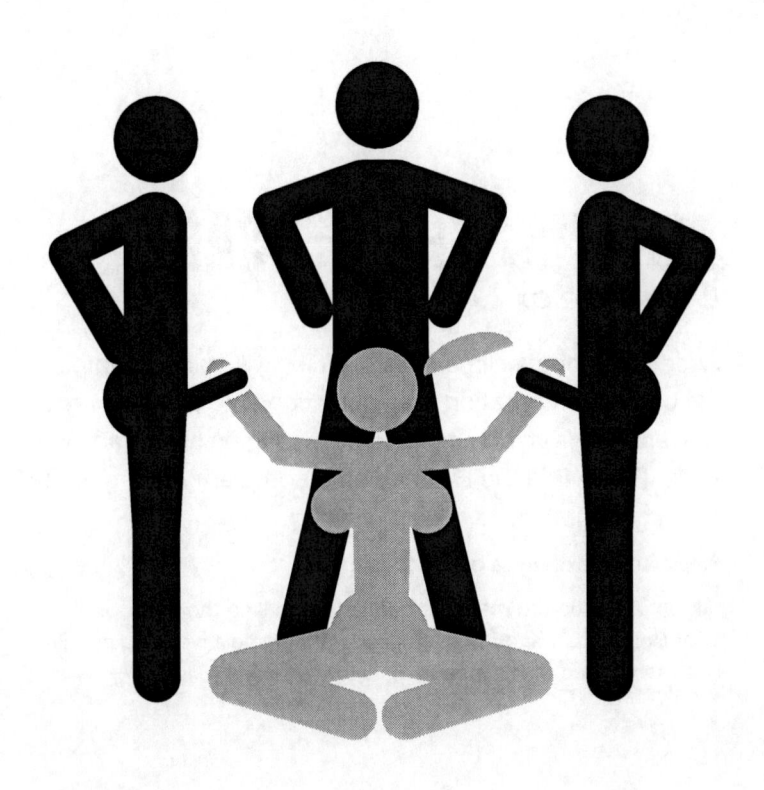

☐ Did It.

Date: ___/___/___ Partner: _____

My Personal Enjoyment (1-10): ☐   My Partner's Enjoyment (1-10): ☐

Comment: _____
_____
_____

PTERODACTYL

PULLING THE E-BRAKE
Consto velox

As the man nears climax, his testicles will pull in towards his body in preparation for ejaculation. The easiest way to prevent him from coming is to gently tug on his retracting balls. Freely Pull the E-Brake until both partners are ready to come together.

Props: Ambidexterity, a gentle touch.

Hot Tip: A gentle tug means a gentle tug, pulling too hard, or "Car Bombing," can turn an aroused partner into a weeping puddle of a man. When that happens, only the terrorists win.

Degree of Difficulty

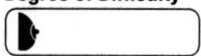

Degree of Nastiness

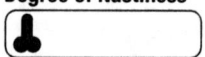

"I've taken the bus my whole life, so giving a soft tug to stop a churning engine is second nature to me. Now we come together every single time."

Anna
Ceramicist
Toronto, Canada

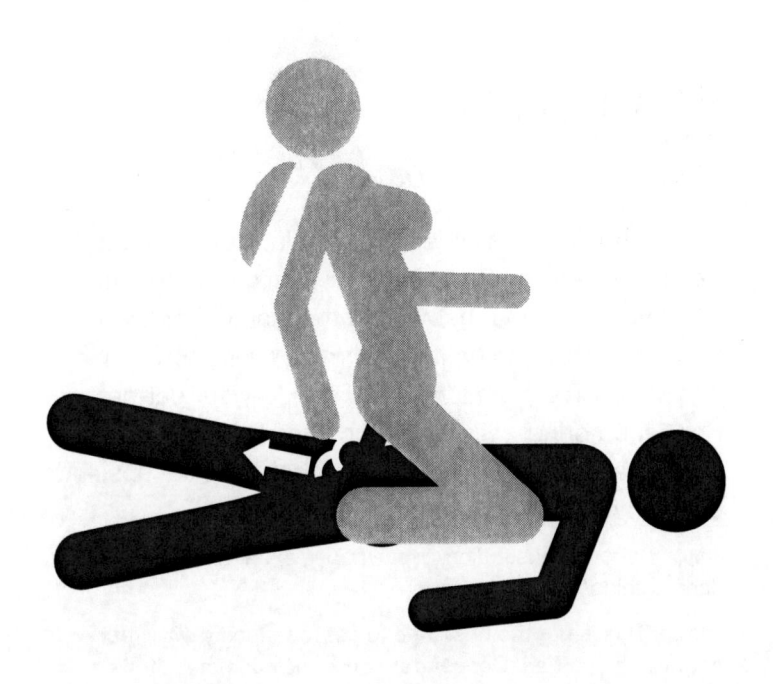

☐ Did It.

Date: ___/___/___   Partner: _____

My Personal
Enjoyment (1-10): ☐   My Partner's
Enjoyment (1-10): ☐

Comment: _____
_____
_____

PULLING THE E-BRAKE

RED WINGS
Cunnilingus cruentus

While some men shy away from having sex while their partner is menstruating, almost all men refrain from going "downtown" during that time of the month. For those brave few willing to do it, performing cunnilingus during menstruation can be a huge turn-on for your partner. Her period brings with it a heightened libido as well as sensual alertness, a time when oral sex feels the absolute best to women.

Props: A strong constitution, tissue paper, extra tampons, dark clothing/sheets.

Hot Tip: This is not the best time to get too friendly with your partner's sex organ. Concentrate on stimulating the clitoris without sucking, lest you have a hankering for a little iron.

Degree of Difficulty

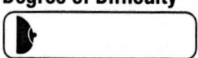

Degree of Nastiness

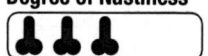

> "My girlfriend always tried to get me to go down on her during her period. When I finally got the nerve to give her some Red Wings, I discovered just how explosive her orgasms can get! What a bloodbath!"
>
> *Edward*
> *Pianist*
> *Forks, Washington*

DIRTY SANCHEZ'S GUIDE TO BUCK NASTY SEX

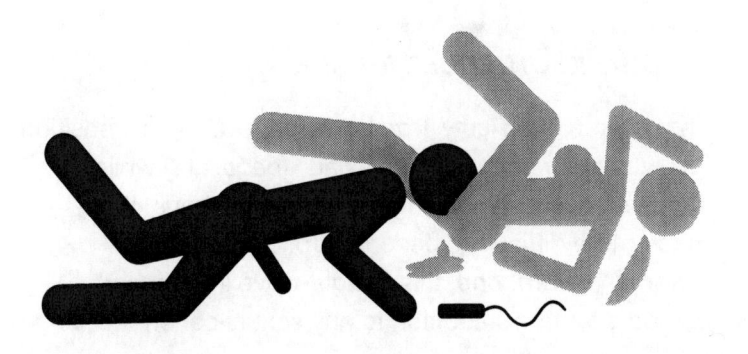

☐ Did It.

Date: ___/___/___   Partner: _____

My Personal
Enjoyment (1-10): ⬜   My Partner's
Enjoyment (1-10): ⬜

Comment: _____
_____
_____

RED WINGS

RUSTY TUBA
Immunda organum femina

The reverse of a Rusty Trombone (page 122), this position involves the man "tossing a salad" (page 112) while simultaneously stimulating his partner's clitoris. While much more difficult to become proficient at than a woman's trombone, this "single-valve instrument" can be a fantastic addition to any sexual canon.

Props: Big brass band record, Mardi Gras beads.

Hot Tip: "Blowing the brass" correctly should end in a full-on female ejaculation in E-flat. The elusive "Dixieland-Double-Drop" can be achieved with a Rusty Tuba, but it's exceptionally rare.

Degree of Difficulty

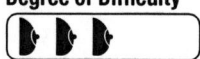

Degree of Nastiness

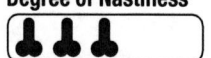

> *"I can't play an instrument to save my life. But when it comes to the Rusty Tuba, I can blow like the best on Bourbon Street."*
>
> *Randy*
> *Salesman*
> *New Orleans, Louisiana*

DIRTY SANCHEZ'S GUIDE TO BUCK NASTY SEX

☐ Did It.

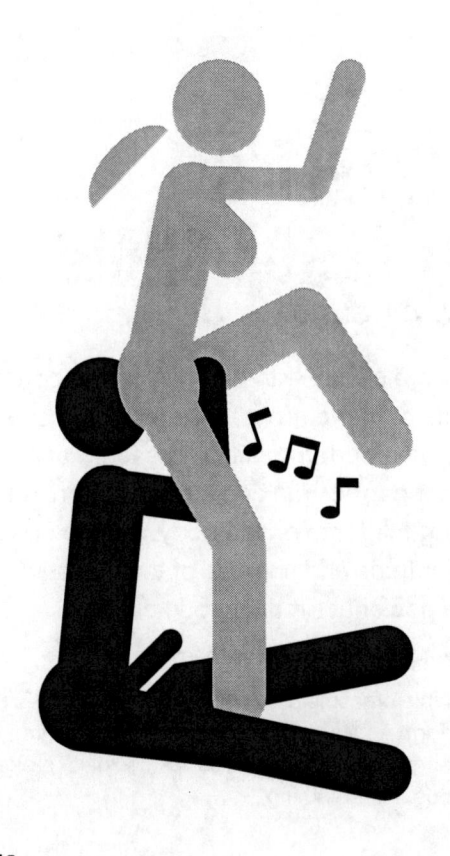

Date: ___/___/___ Partner: _____

My Personal
Enjoyment (1-10): ☐

My Partner's
Enjoyment (1-10): ☐

Comment: _____
_____
_____

RUSTY TUBA

SEA WORLD'S SIX O'CLOCK SHOW
Balaena percutio

Shortly before climax with the man on the bottom, the woman lifts off her partner while making majestic whale calls. She then performs a full "breach," launching off of her spent partner, making a quarter turn in the air and landing full-force on his body. If done correctly, the spectacular force and surprise of the maneuver should result in a powerful simultaneous climax.

Props: A bucket of fish, spyglass, harpoon.

Hot Tip: Multiple orgasms are possible if the woman is physically able to perform a "Moby Dick," repeatedly punishing her partner with vicious, hull-crushing blows. Once satisfied, make sure he's still conscious and breathing.

Degree of Difficulty

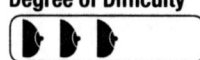

Degree of Nastiness

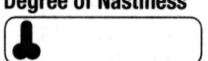

"Marge weighs in around three bills, so when she Sea Worlds me, it's like Shamu got angry. If it's too much, I ask her to give me a little warning, you know, a 'thar she blows' or something."

Christopher
Shopkeeper
Nantucket, Massachusetts

DIRTY SANCHEZ'S GUIDE TO BUCK NASTY SEX

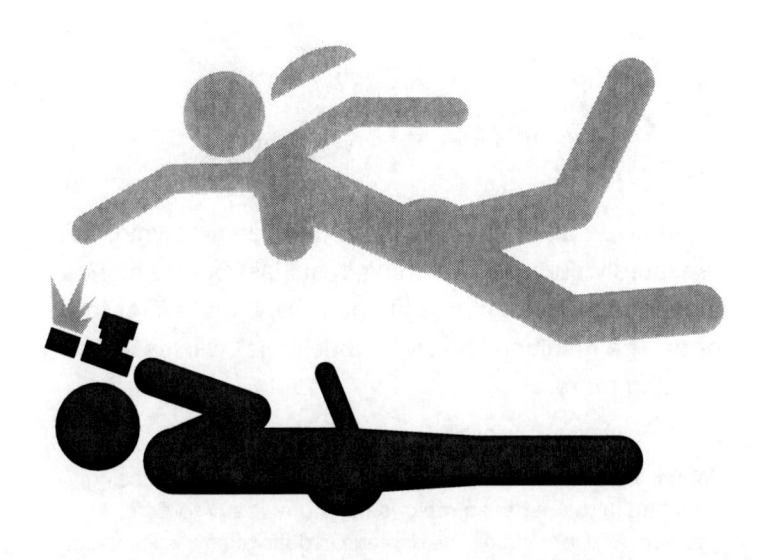

☐ Did It.

Date: ___/___/___   Partner: _____

My Personal Enjoyment (1-10): ☐   My Partner's Enjoyment (1-10): ☐

Comment: _____
_____
_____

SEA WORLD'S SIX O'CLOCK SHOW

SPEED BAGGIN'
Dolor valde

As the woman rides her partner in reverse cowgirl, she repeatedly punches him in his testicles. Before he has a chance to orgasm, she jumps off and makes for the door. The resulting "black 'n' blue balls" will leave him wanting more.

Props: Practice bag, gloves.

Hot Tip: Keep your guard up—only a select few men like being punched in the nads, so make sure you're ready to defend yourself. And remember, the damage is done after a few knocks, so deliver them rapidly and move out of the way.

Degree of Difficulty

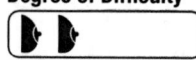

Degree of Nastiness

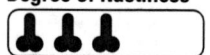

> *"Talk about 'sting like a bee.' This was like 'sting like a box jellyfish attached to a shark.' I think Holyfield got off easy getting his ear bit off."*
>
> Carlton
> Farm worker
> Jackson Hole, Wyoming

☐ Did It.

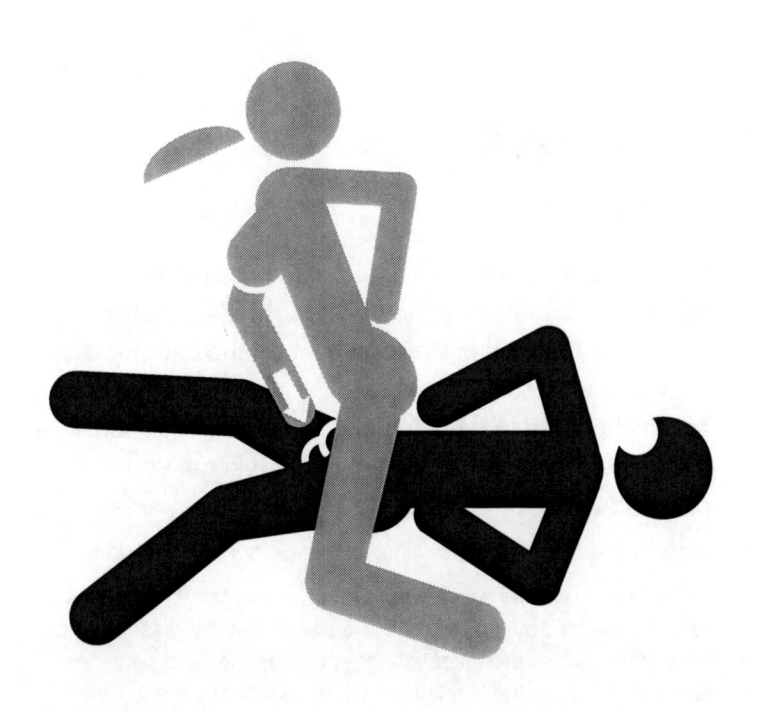

Date: ___/___/___   Partner: _____

My Personal
Enjoyment (1-10): ☐   My Partner's
Enjoyment (1-10): ☐

Comment: _____
_____
_____

SPEED BAGGIN'

SUPERMAN
Deussapien

A classic role-playing finish, the man pulls out of doggy style and ejaculates between his partner's shoulder blades. He then takes the top sheet off the bed and slaps it onto her wet, sticky back, creating a long, flowing cape. Take a little time to have fun and run around the house as crime-fighting superheroes — it might just get you ready for round two!

Props: Phone booth, arch criminal, extensive comic collection.

Hot Tip: Watery semen is everyone's kryptonite in this situation, as it's quickly absorbed by the cloth. To ensure the densest finish possible, make sure you've taken a couple days off from sex and complete your Superman on the first love-making session of the day.

Degree of Difficulty

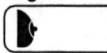

Degree of Nastiness

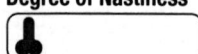

"It's frickin' amazing — with some boots, a girdle and a tiara, my girlfriend is instantly transformed from an average gal to Superwoman herself. It never gets old."

Dave
Collector
Flagstaff, Arizona

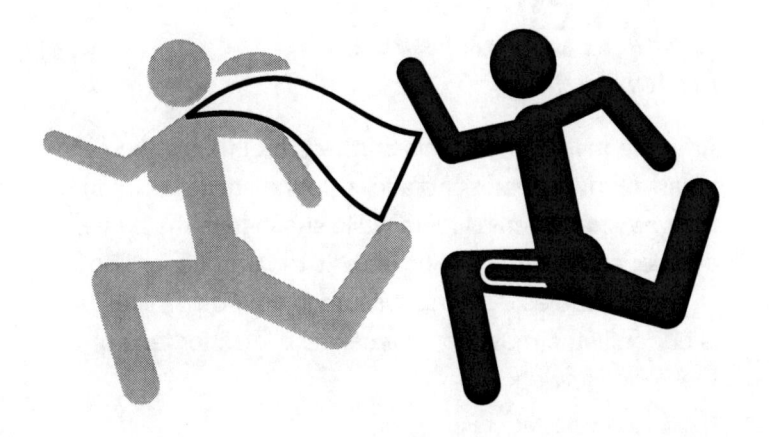

☐ Did It.

Date: ___/___/___   Partner: _____

My Personal Enjoyment (1-10): ☐   My Partner's Enjoyment (1-10): ☐

Comment: _____
_____
_____

SUPERMAN

THANKSGIVING TURKEY STUFF
Fartor cena

After the man comes in his partner's mouth, the woman takes a turkey baster and sucks up the seed. The man then gets down on all fours while she inserts the baster and squeezes out the juice into his rectum. According to recent studies, "getting roasted in your own juices" is currently the most popular sexual climax for fans of the Food Network.

Props: Turkey baster, cranberry sauce.

Hot Tip: The hotter the juice, the more tender the meat. Make sure to have the props on hand before he finishes; letting the sperm cool before insertion is not only less arousing, it can be downright uncomfortable too.

Degree of Difficulty

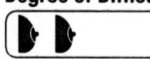

Degree of Nastiness

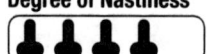

> "I always squirt a little lemon or lime into my mouth before grabbing for the baster. Not only does it freshen the semen, it adds a thrilling little zest for him!"
>
> *Bertha*
> *Stay-at-home mom*
> *Miami Beach, Florida*

DIRTY SANCHEZ'S GUIDE TO BUCK NASTY SEX

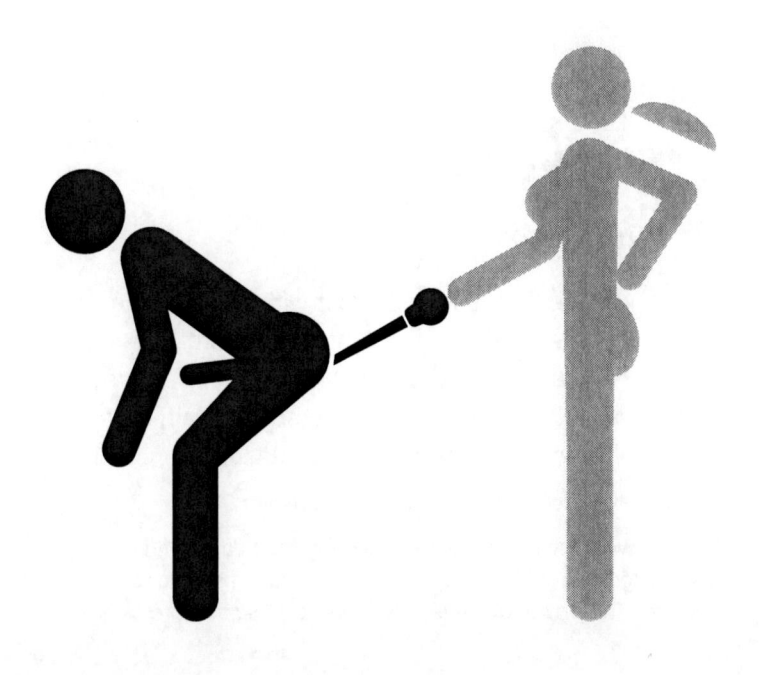

☐ Did It.

Date: ___/___/___   Partner: _____

My Personal
Enjoyment (1-10): ☐   My Partner's
Enjoyment (1-10): ☐

Comment: _____
_____
_____

THANKSGIVING TURKEY STUFF

THE EXORCIST
Sanctus vomito

As the woman finishes her partner with oral sex, the man pushes his erect penis deeper into her mouth. The sudden shot of hot semen combined with a tonsil-tickling deep throat should make the woman projectile vomit. It's a messy end, to say the least, but spectacular nonetheless.

Props: Holy water, bucket, towel, stain remover.

Hot Tip: Everyone loves a priestly fantasy from time to time. Try giving her a little thrill by proclaiming something along the lines of "The Power of Christ Compels You!" just before climax.

Degree of Difficulty

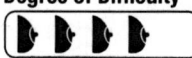

Degree of Nastiness

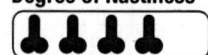

"I'm really not into exercising, but exorcising is the best way to lose weight."
Debra
Telemarketer
Fort Lauderdale, Florida

DIRTY SANCHEZ'S GUIDE TO BUCK NASTY SEX

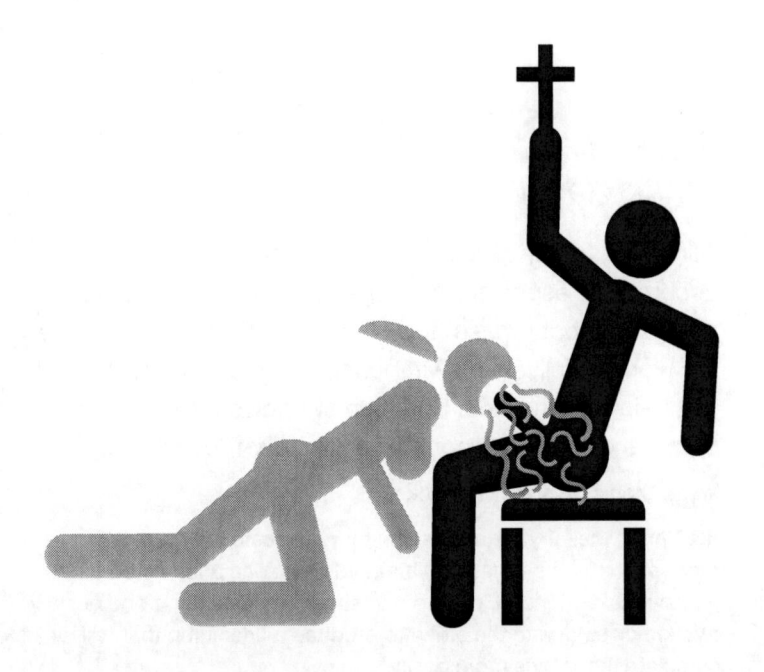

☐ Did It.

Date: ___/___/___   Partner: _____

My Personal Enjoyment (1-10): ☐   My Partner's Enjoyment (1-10): ☐

Comment: _____
_____
_____

THE EXORCIST

THE LAST UNICORN
Equus magus

Climaxing together is not the easiest sexual feat to accomplish, especially for a premature man who leaves his partner without orgasm too often. After the man has come, the woman delivers a swift punch to the crown of his head, just below the hairline. She then straddles the inflamed bump and "rides the horn" to a rainbow-filled climax.

Props: Magic crystals, ice pack.

Hot Tip: As the fairytale states, the more delicate the horn, the more powerful the orgasm. Instead of delivering a full-fisted blow to the man's forehead, the woman should try extending one or two knuckles during the strike to produce a finer lump that will stimulate the clitoris more easily.

Degree of Difficulty

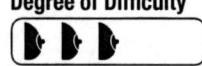

Degree of Nastiness

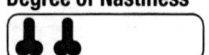

> *"My boyfriend lasted about 30 seconds every time we made love. For one year I didn't get off—it almost ended our relationship. But when my sister told me about The Last Unicorn, it revolutionized everything. He says I'm worth the chronic headaches. Now that's love."*
>
> Lili
> Stylist
> Denver, Colorado

DIRTY SANCHEZ'S GUIDE TO BUCK NASTY SEX

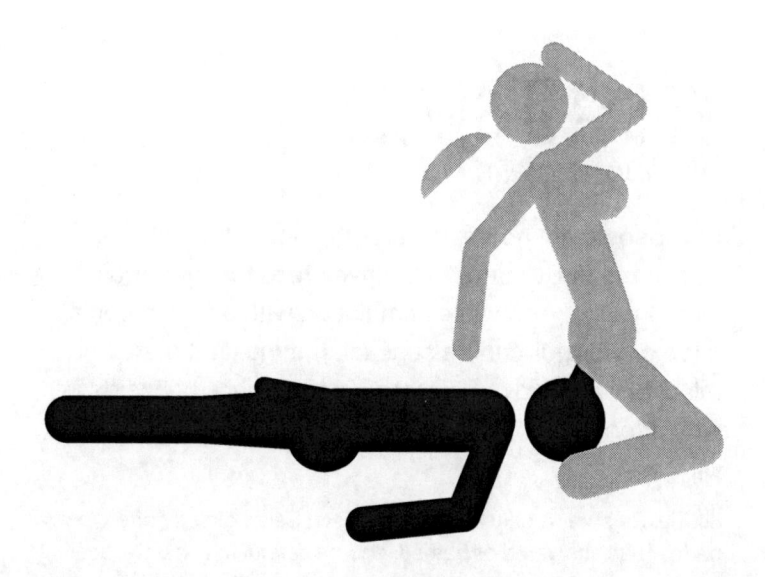

☐ Did It.

Date: ___/___/___   Partner: _____

My Personal
Enjoyment (1-10): ☐   My Partner's
Enjoyment (1-10): ☐

Comment: _____
_____
_____

THE LAST UNICORN

TOSSED SALAD
Analingus classicus

Few people acknowledge that the rim of the anus is one of the body's most sensitive areas for men and women alike. And while stimulation with a finger, penis, dildo or vibrator can be sensual, the most intimate and mind-blowing way of pleasuring a partner's backside is with a tongue.

Props: Soap.

Hot Tip: Be sure to only attempt a Tossed Salad directly after your partner has showered or bathed, and be careful to avoid the act if you have any open cuts or sores on your mouth.

Degree of Difficulty

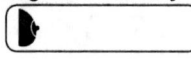

Degree of Nastiness

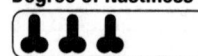

> *"I would never marry a man who refuses to eat a little ass."*
> Anon.
> Overheard on the MTA
> Queens, New York

DIRTY SANCHEZ'S GUIDE TO BUCK NASTY SEX

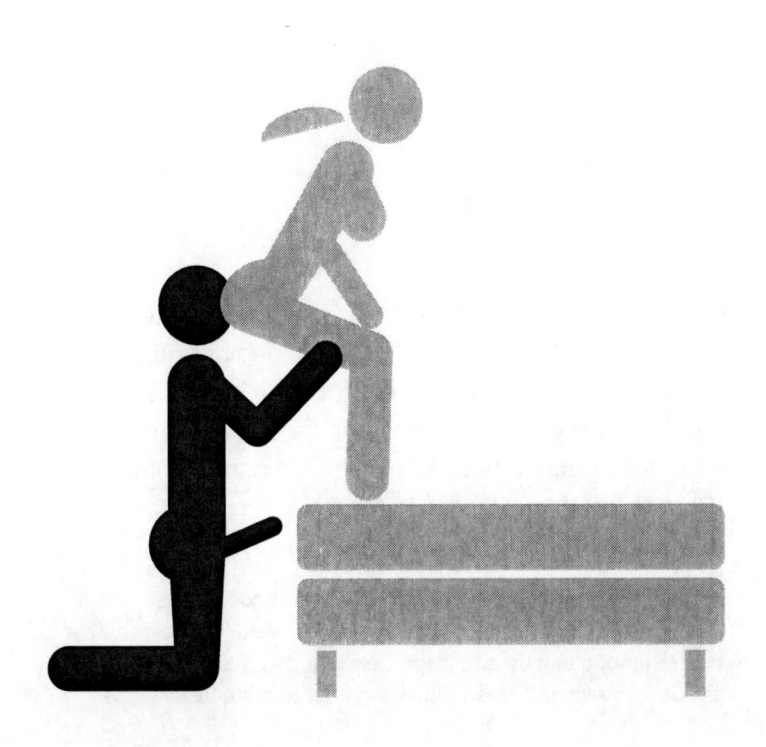

☐ Did It.

Date: ___/___/___   Partner: _____

My Personal Enjoyment (1-10): ☐   My Partner's Enjoyment (1-10): ☐

Comment: _____
_____
_____

TOSSED SALAD

TRIPLE DIP
Tria mihi

The ultimate goal for most men, the vagina-anus-mouth hat trick is not easily done. The man begins with slow, tender intercourse before gently inserting his member into his partner's anus. On the verge of climax, the man pulls out and heads north for his partner's mouth. What happens next is up to the fates.

Props: Lube, douche, enema, mouthwash.

Hot Tip: A good washing can mean the difference between a full triple dip and a lame two-layered bean dip. Make your preparations beforehand, clean up and clean deep. And above all, try talking about your plans, instead of leaving it up to chance.

Degree of Difficulty

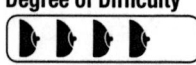

Degree of Nastiness

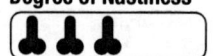

> "I never was into watching porn like my husband, but I learned a lot about the Triple Dip from his favorite movies, and I gotta say, it's a very intimate way to have him."
>
> *Tracy*
> *Makeup artist*
> *Hollywood, California*

DIRTY SANCHEZ'S GUIDE TO BUCK NASTY SEX

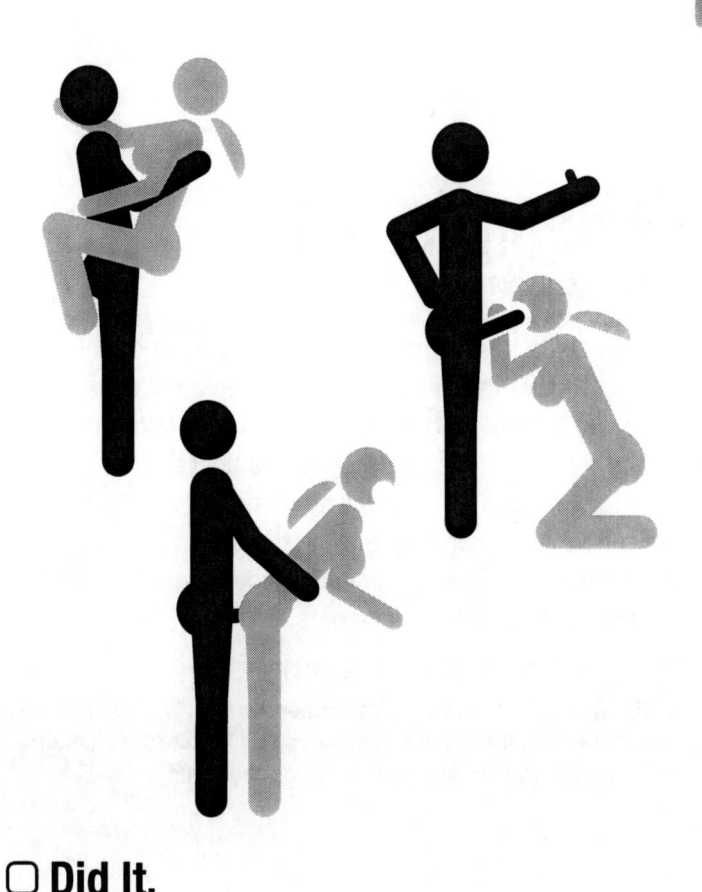

☐ Did It.

Date: ___/___/___   Partner: _____

My Personal Enjoyment (1-10): ☐   My Partner's Enjoyment (1-10): ☐

Comment: _____
_____
_____

TRIPLE DIP

VAMPIRE TEA BAG
Esurio cruentus

Foreplay with the woman on her period can be as fun as it is intimidating. If both partners decide to have some messy sex, begin with this fun move. With the woman spread eagle, the man grabs her tampon string between his incisors and delicately pulls it out, letting the engorged cotton slap him on the chin, spilling the blood down his neck and chest. A little Edward-on-Bella role play can take over from here.

Props: Used tampon, dark sheets, *Twilight* box set.

Hot Tip: The fresher the blood, the better the play. Nothing kills a vampire fantasy like a crusty tampon, so make sure the woman's flow is recent and strong before initiating the Vampire Tea Bag.

Degree of Difficulty

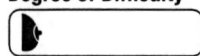

Degree of Nastiness

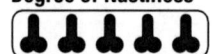

"When my boyfriend does this, it's totally like having sex with a real vampire. Hot. Like Edward Cullen hot!"

Brianna
Student
Reno, Nevada

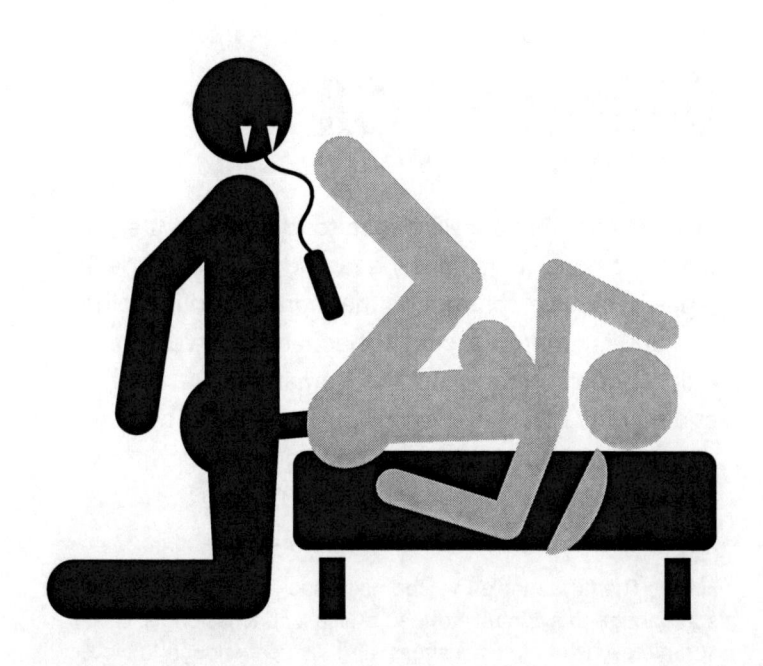

☐ Did It.

Date: ___/___/___   Partner: _____

My Personal
Enjoyment (1-10): ☐   My Partner's
Enjoyment (1-10): ☐

Comment: _____
_____
_____

VAMPIRE TEA BAG

Donkey Punch
Retrocopulation inflictum

The man delivers a swift punch to the back of the woman's head while finishing in doggy-style, triggering a pelvic-muscle contraction that tightens both vagina and anus and dramatically enhances the male orgasm. Wildly popular throughout the Roman Empire, the taut ending of the Donkey Punch was once described by the philosopher Anguitentis as "a boa constrictor swallowing a baby bull."

Props: Hand wrap, ice pack, painkillers, smelling salts.

Hot Tip: The fashionable EverTec AssSmack boxing gloves are soft enough to avoid unintended bruises, concussions and complete loss of consciousness, and discreet enough to hide anywhere in the bedroom.

Degree of Difficulty
4

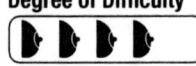

Degree of Nastiness
3

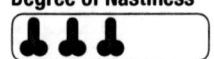

"The slight concussion is a small price to pay for not having to do any Kegel exercises."
Princess
Hotel manager
Kailua, Hawaii

DIRTY SANCHEZ'S GUIDE TO BUCK NASTY SEX

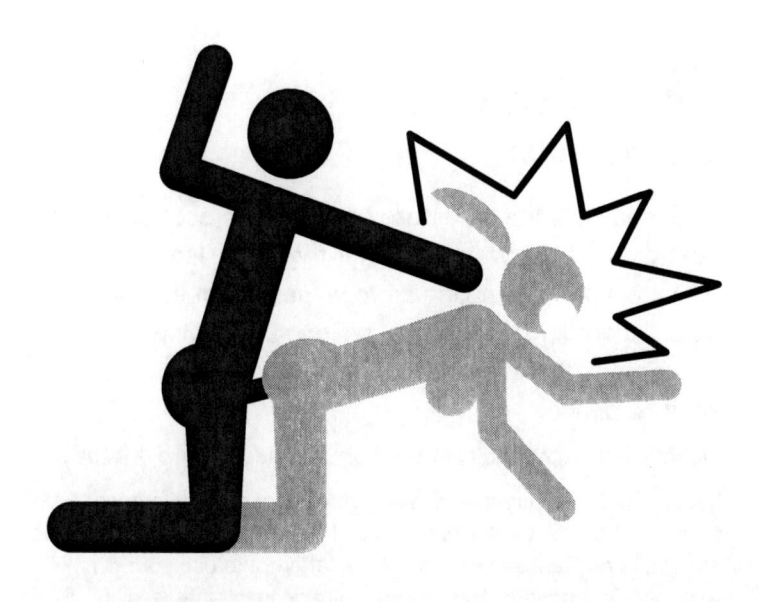

☐ Did It.

Date: ___/___/___   Partner: _____

My Personal Enjoyment (1-10): ☐   My Partner's Enjoyment (1-10): ☐

Comment: _____
_____
_____

DONKEY PUNCH

NEW DELHI DOT
Macula fecum

After anal sex, the man pulls out his still-erect penis and gently pokes the woman on her forehead, leaving a delicate stain resembling a brown version of the Indian *bindi*. According to tradition, as long as the New Delhi Dot is worn, the woman will have remarkable fortune and spiritual peace.

Props: A sumptuous Indian, Nepali or Bangladeshi meal, Kleenex.

Hot Tip: There's a very subtle, but highly noticeable, difference between the New Dehli Dot and the classic Dirty Unibrow. Chances are you're no Ganesha, so before you attempt to use your "trunk" to apply a bean *bindi*, practice your aim on inanimate, easily sterilized objects.

Degree of Difficulty

Degree of Nastiness

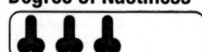

> "We always planned on going to India for our honeymoon, but our finances got wiped out in the recession. When Stan gave me my first New Delhi Dot, I felt something spiritual, a connection from West to East. It's not India, but it is something close."
>
> *Diana Sunshine*
> *Yoga instructor*
> *Oakland, California*

☐ Did It.

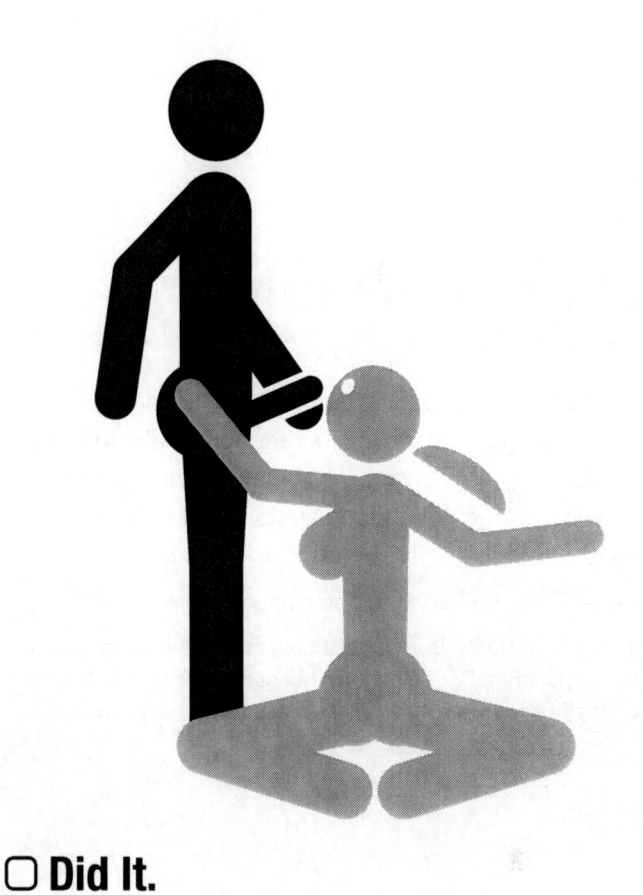

Date: ___/___/___   Partner: _____

My Personal
Enjoyment (1-10): ☐

My Partner's
Enjoyment (1-10): ☐

Comment: _____
_____
_____

NEW DELHI DOT

RUSTY TROMBONE
Immunda organum

The woman kneels behind the man and "tosses a salad" (see page 112) while simultaneously giving him a handjob. A classic position popular among music aficionados, to the voyeuristic bystander it looks like a vigorous trombone solo.

Props: Knee pads, up-tempo jazz soundtrack.

Hot Tip: The best Rusty Trombone should end with male ejaculation ("Blowing a Coltrane"), defecation ("Mingus to the Mouth") or the exceptionally rare duel discharge ("Dixieland Double Drop").

Degree of Difficulty

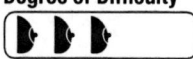

Degree of Nastiness

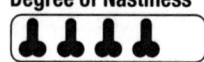

"The best notes hit you smack in the face and make you smile."

Scarlett
Music teacher
Long Island City, New York

DIRTY SANCHEZ'S GUIDE TO BUCK NASTY SEX

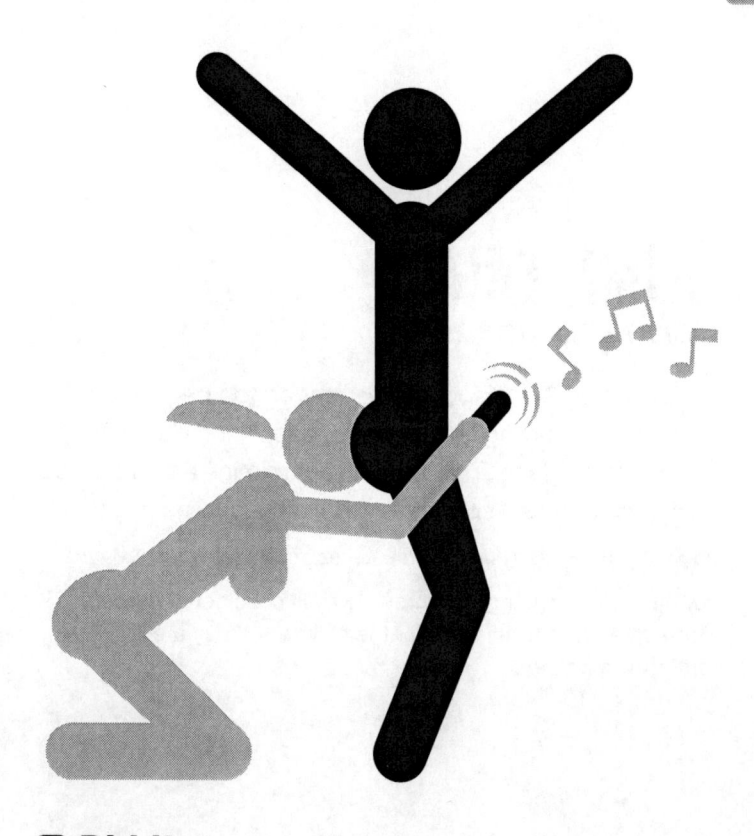

☐ Did It.

Date: ___/___/___   Partner: _____

My Personal
Enjoyment (1-10): ☐

My Partner's
Enjoyment (1-10): ☐

Comment: _____
_____
_____

RUSTY TROMBONE

DUMP TRUCK
Quisquiliae liberatio

While in the 69 position, the partner on top begins to sit upright while saying "beep, beep, beep" and defecating on the other's face. This sensual act mimics a dump truck raising its bed and spilling its dirty, dirty load on a landfill.

Props: Charlie Sheen *and* Emilio Estevez, mob protection, overalls.

Hot Tip: Not everything you throw away is considered garbage. Remember to recycle. Do it for the children—they are tomorrow's future.

Degree of Difficulty

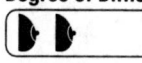

Degree of Nastiness

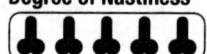

"There's always been something about sanitation for me. You know, something romantic. The way the mob controls it, the way they come around so regularly. I don't know, it looks carefree. Nice. They make a lot of money too."

Trevor
Computer programmer
Trenton, New Jersey

☐ Did It.

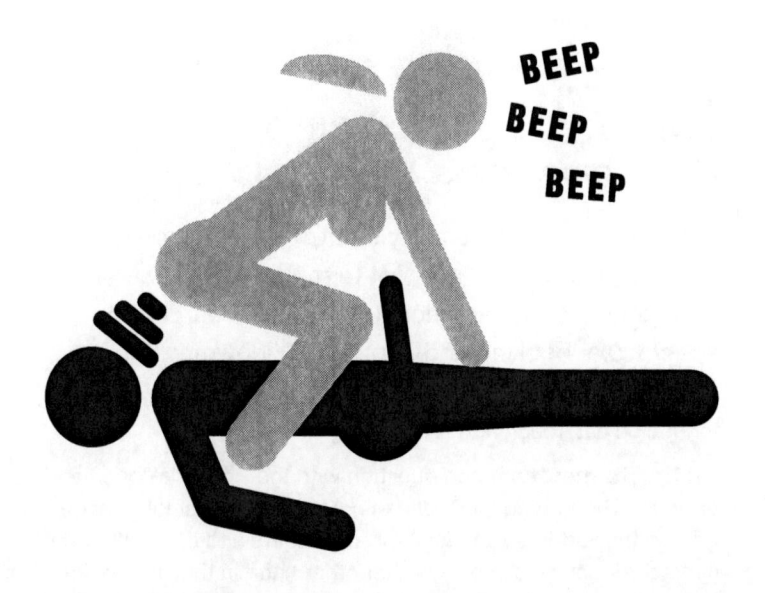

Date: ___/___/___   Partner: _____

My Personal
Enjoyment (1-10): [   ]   My Partner's
Enjoyment (1-10): [   ]

Comment: _____
_____
_____

DUMP TRUCK

RODEO
Concumbo bovus

Following the surprise entry of a group of friends (or relatives) mid-coitus, attempt to maintain intercourse for eight seconds. Additional points are awarded for spectacular bucking and impressive showmanship.

Props: Acquaintances, closet or other clandestine locale, timer, ten-gallon hat, rough rider belt buckle.

Hot Tip: The most common question with the Rodeo is "one hand or two?" The traditional Rodeo encourages a firm single-handed grip on the "udders" (breasts) for male riders and the "soft horns" (testes) for cowgirls. Now get that other hand in the air and ride like the wind.

Degree of Difficulty

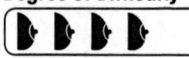

Degree of Nastiness

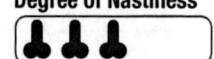

> *"My favorite Rodeo is the one you do with the whole family."*
> Michael
> Musician
> Flint, Michigan

☐ Did It.

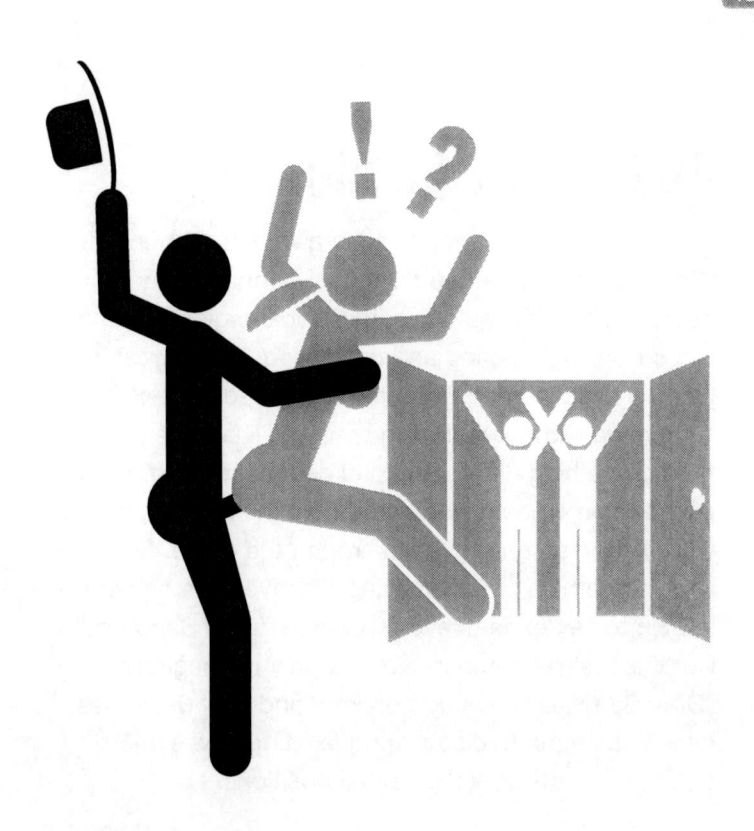

Date: ___/___/___   Partner: _____

My Personal Enjoyment (1-10): ☐   My Partner's Enjoyment (1-10): ☐

Comment: _____
_____
_____

RODEO

ABOUT THE AUTHOR

A respected dentist who lived in a wealthy suburb of Cincinnati and attended his local Methodist church every Sunday, the author of this book originally found sex surprisingly boring and unfulfilling. And it wasn't just the Ohio women. He often described his sex life as "cumming without really orgasming." Then one day he tried something different and experienced an intensely pleasurable orgasm—he had drawn the handlebars that would soon spread to faces around the globe. As he informed others of his amazing discovery, he became known to sex experts everywhere as "Dirty Sanchez." But this first patented move was only the beginning. "Dirty Sanchez" gave up dentistry and now dedicates himself full-time to discovering exciting new eye-popping, heart-stopping sexual positions.